ANTI-INFLAMMATORY
DIET COOKBOOK FOR
BEGINNERS

1000 Easy and Delicious Anti-inflammatory Recipes with 28-Day Meal Plan

to Reduce Inflammation and Lead a Healthy Lifestyle.

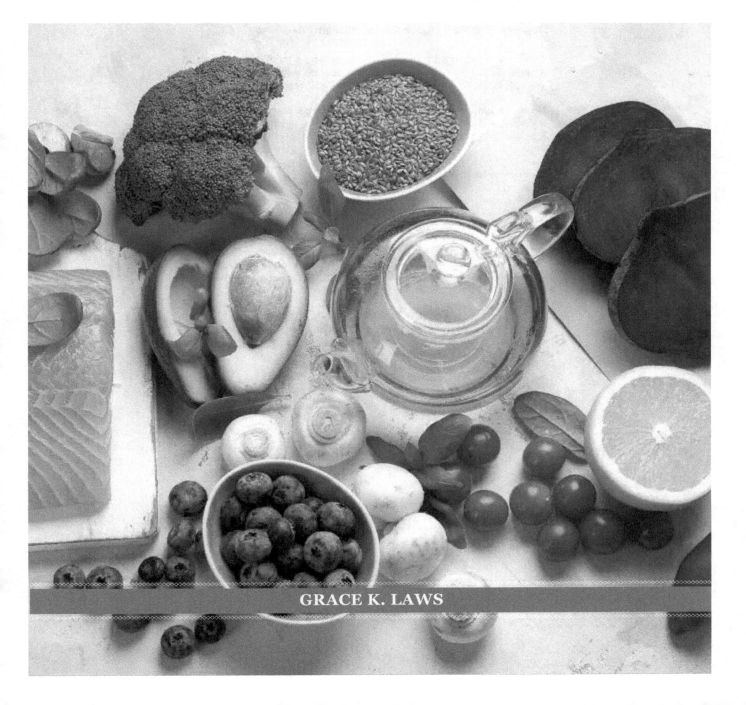

GRACE K. LAWS

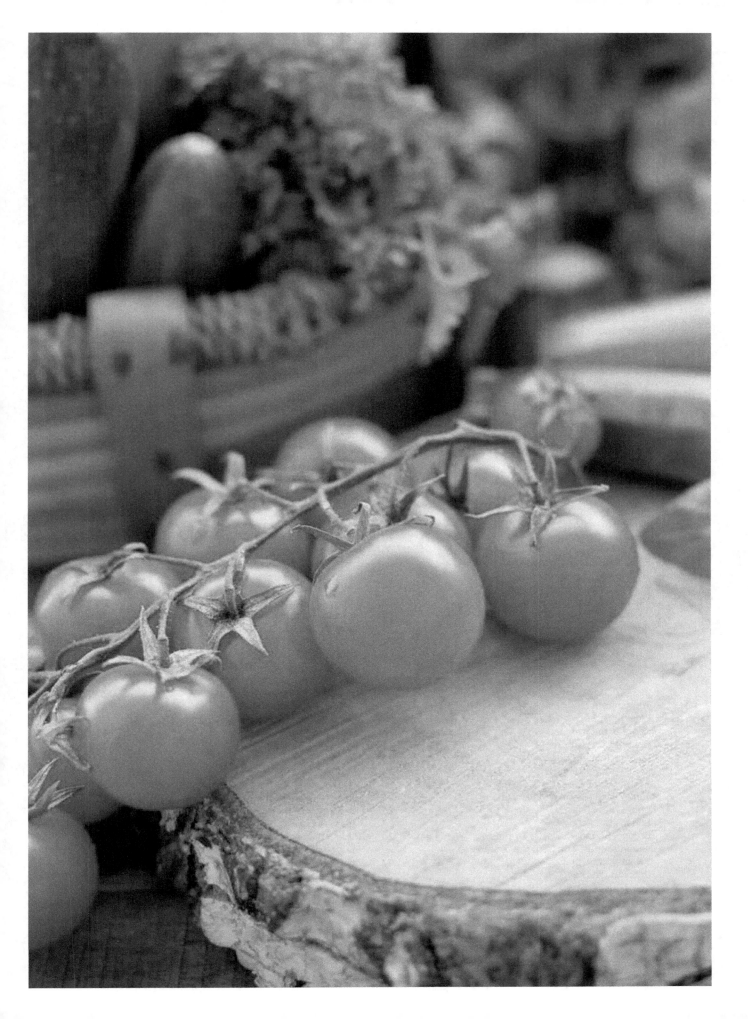

Table of Contents

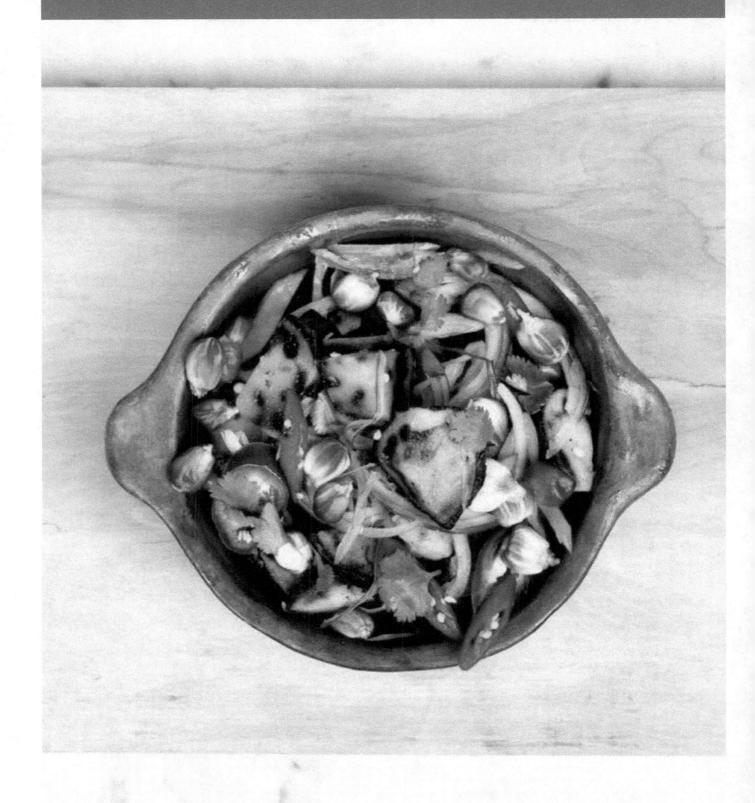

There was this very meaningful illustration that I saw the other day. In that illustration, there were two doors, one led to the doctor and it had a long line, the other one was about changing lifestyle and no one was going towards it. We want the problem to be solved but we never want to figure out the reason behind the problem. It is reported that approximately 678,000 people in the United States die each year from unhealthy diets and that diabetes is one of the leading causes of amputations. Your body showing inflammation signs does not always mean you have a serious disease or you need medications, sometimes all your body is asking for is change.

I am here with this guideline to help people realize the importance of an anti-inflammatory diet as what you eat makes you what you are, healthy or unhealthy. Inflammation is a marker of disease and premature aging. If you are fighting inflammation, you are fighting several diseases and aging your body considerably. In this article, we will learn what inflammation is and why it's dangerous. We will also meet foods that cause inflammation and cook delicious anti-inflammatory recipes that can help you reduce the risk of cancer, heart disease, diabetes, depression, and even Alzheimer's.

Chapter 1
Basics of Inflammation

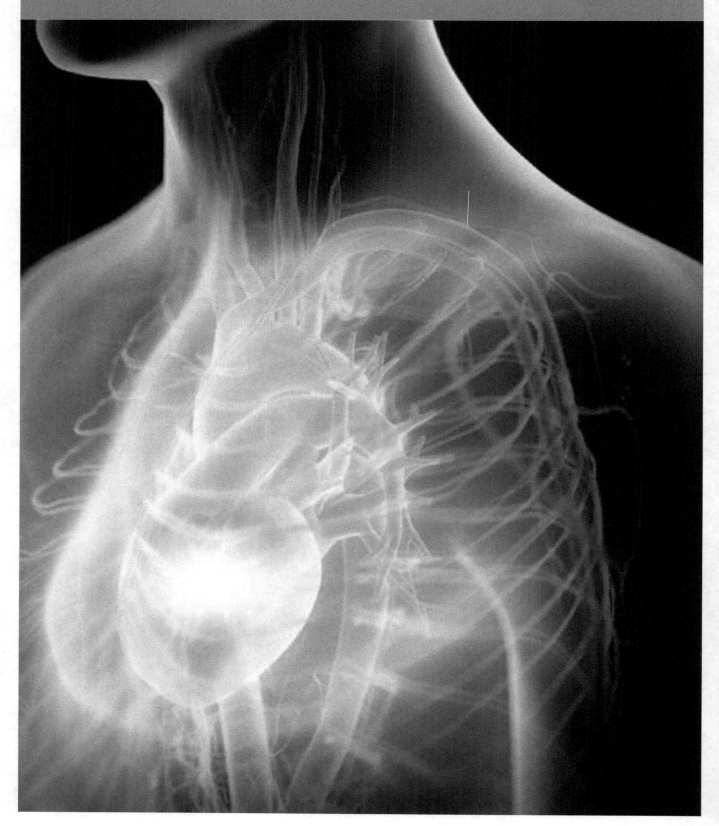

What is inflammation?

Inflammation is your body's natural response to any injury and infection in your body. Inflammation has two types; Acute and Chronic Inflammation. Inflammation is a two-sided coin; it is both good and bad. On one hand, it helps your body defend itself from infections and on the other hand chronic inflammation can lead to diseases.

ACUTE INFLAMMATION:

Acute inflammation is a sudden and short-term response of the immune system to injuries like cuts. It is less severe and heals over time.

CHRONIC INFLAMMATION:

Chronic inflammation is prolonged inflammation that occurs due to a toxin in the body like smoke from cigarettes that causes lung diseases. An unhealthy diet is a huge contributor to chronic inflammation. For example, high sugar levels can cause diabetes which currently there is no cure for and is only controlled by diet and exercise.

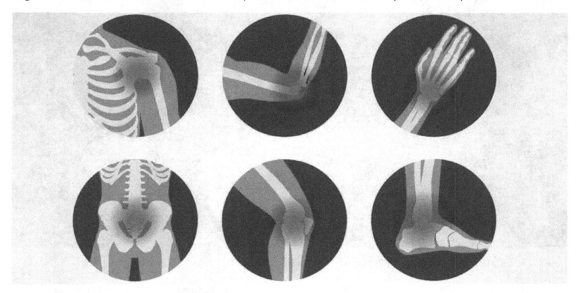

What Causes Chronic Inflammation?

A hypothesis has been deducted based on a few research studies that show a correlation between certain factors and inflammation. Some of those factors include:

ANTIBIOTICS

Antibiotic misuse and overuse can lead to chronic inflammation, which has been linked to alterations of the micro-biome. How inflammation causes this alteration is still a mystery.

ENVIRONMENTAL FACTORS

Factors like air pollution, cigarette smoke, industrial waste, and polluted water can lead to chronic inflammation.

What is the Role of Diet in Inflammation?

As we mentioned earlier, what you eat can lead to chronic inflammation like Gastrointestinal problems and diseases. In today's world, people want everything as quickly and easy as possible and unfortunately this carries over into our eating habits as well. We prefer going out instead of cooking, or buying quick frozen easy meals rather than fresh healthier options. Junk food is the best friend of this generation.

Processed foods usually contain high levels of sugar, sodium, ands fats. All these things make the food taste great, but in return can cause health issues such as high cholesterol. People often face a loth of health problems but fail to find the source. At times even turning to medical professionals returns no diagnosis because the issues are diet related.

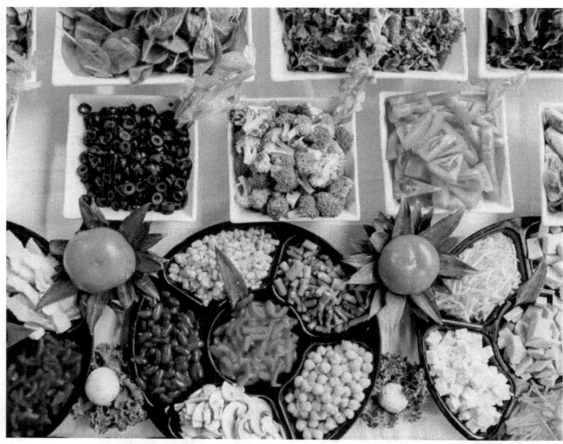

How Do You Know You Have Inflammation?

Two tings can help to diagnose chronic inflammation. The first are symptoms which we will list below and the second is a medical test known as hsCRP.

Symptoms of chronic inflammation include:

- Mental health issues
- Mood swings
- Weight gain
- Weight loss
- Insomnia
- Gastrointestinal problems, like constipation, acid reflux, diarrhea, etc

THE EFFECT OF CHRONIC INFLAMMATION ON THE BODY'S FUNCTION:

The human body has a natural mechanism to cope with or eliminate harmful toxin material from the body. The human body has a natural mechanism to cope with or eliminate harmful toxic materials in the body. But if the number of free radicals is in excess in the human body it generates oxidative stress that can cause chronic problems which in return increases free-radical production and decreases the mechanism of anti-oxidants. Antioxidants are of two types

- Naturally produced in the body.
- Externally supplied through supplements and food.

Another crucial part of the human body is the digestive system and its health is determined by what goes into it from the outside. A high quantity of junk food can lower the digestion process which can lead to bloating as junk food does not contain the enzyme that natural and cooked food has.

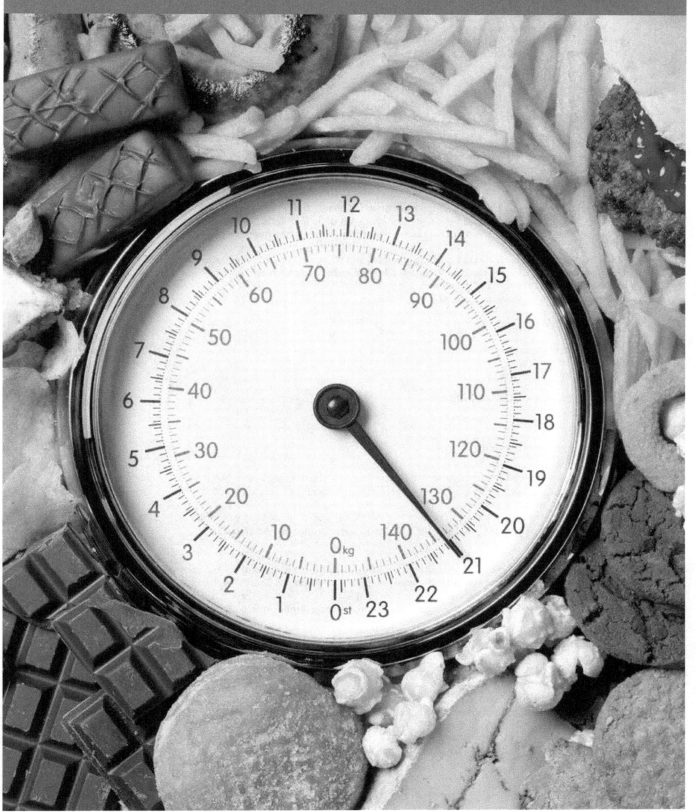

Chapter 2
Start your Anti-Inflammatory Diet

Foods that cause Inflammation

Now that we have established that diet is one of the main factors that can contribute to inflammation, let us look at the food that can cause inflammation.

DIETARY SUGAR:

According to a study, sugar intake can increase the chances of developing breast cancer. A lot of people have this misconception that sugar intake can only cause diabetes which is not valid. In fact with diabetes, it can also increase tumor chances and some studies found out high sugar level increase triglyceride in the body which leads to the thickening of arteries.

TRANS-FAT:

There are two kinds of trans-fat one that is naturally produced in cattle through bacteria and a controlled intake does not cause it to be harmful. But the other kind, known as Artificial trans fat is highly dangerous for health, as they are prepared by the addition of hydrogen in unsaturated oils to increase its shelf life.
Trans fats increase bad cholesterol and decrease good cholesterol, Severly harming the heart.

SEED AND VEGETABLE OILS:

People might think seed and vegetable oils are good for health, but studies found out that some oils from seeds and vegetables that are high in Omega-6 contents are not good for health. Omega-6 and Omega-3 are important fatty acids, the body needs them in a certain amount through diet as the human body itself can not produce them.

In the beginning, humans used to consume omega-6 and omega-3 in a certain ratio but with time the ratio shifted drastically from 1:1 to 20:1, and scientists have hypothesized too much omega-6 consumption as compared to omega-3 can cause chronic inflammation.
It can cause obesity, bowel disease, and heart disease.

OILS TO AVOID:
- Corn oil
- Sunflower oil
- Sesame oil
- Peanut oil

OILS THAT ARE GOOD FOR HEALTH:
- Coconut oil
- Olive oil

REFINED CARBOHYDRATES

Not all Carbohydrates are bad for the body, carbohydrates high in fiber prove to provide health benefits. But refined carbohydrates that have the majority of the fibers removed can lead to bacteria in the inflammatory gut that can cause obesity and bowel disease.
Refined carbohydrates, such as white bread and pasta, are also a major source of inflammation. These foods are high in sugar and can contribute to weight gain, blood sugar problems, and diabetes.

ALCOHOL

Excessive alcohol consumption can lead to a "leaky gut", where bacterias and toxins leak from the intestinal wall into the bloodstream and can cause inflammation. Each time alcohol is filtered by the liver, some liver cells die in the process, and the liver can regenerate new cells. But excessive consumptions increase the ratio of cell death to the ratio of cell reproduction which can cause liver damage, as a famous quote says " excess of everything is bad"

PROCESSED MEATS

Processed meats for example bacon, sausage, and deli meat, are abundant in saturated fat and sodium. These nutrients can increase inflammation in the body and lead to health problems such as heart disease and stroke.

FAST FOOD

Fast food is another type of food that can cause inflammation. Fast food is often high in fat, salt, and calories, and can contribute to weight gain. Fast food can also be high in sugar and refined carbohydrates, which can increase blood sugar levels and lead to diabetes.

SUGARY DRINKS

Sugary drinks such as soda and energy drinks are also major sources of inflammation. These drinks are high in sugar and can contribute to weight gain, heart disease, and diabetes.

Anti-Inflammatory Food

AVOCADOS

Eating avocados has proven to have a healthy effect, A study found out that eating hamburgers with avocados decreased the inflammatory response as they contain anti-oxidants and mono-unsaturated fats.
Four ounces of avocado have 227 calories, 9-gram fibers, 3 grams of protein, and 21 grams of fat, of which 75% are healthy mono and polyunsaturated fats.
Some other benefits of avocados:

- Improves digestion.
- Improves liver health.
- Heals arthritis.

DARK CHOCOLATE

Dark chocolate is the yummiest anti-inflammatory diet as it is full of antioxidants. It is suitable for numerous body organs and functions. Flavanols found in cocoa have been shown to lower blood pressure, improve blood flow, wrestle cell damage, and avert blood clots.

Dark chocolate with 70 or more percent of cocoa content improves cardiac health by improving arterial blood flow.

- Eggs

Known as the perfect food by the doctors, there is no healthy diet that does not contain eggs in it. Eggs contain carotenoids zeaxanthin and lutein (both beneficial for vision), and they also contain choline which is good for the brain and heart. Eggs contain vitamin D, protein, and vitamin B, eggs have been shown to provide numerous health benefits:

- Healthy heart.
- Promote good cholesterol.
- Lowers Triglycerides.
- Affordable.

FISH

Cold-water fish have a good amount of unsaturated fatty acids and low mercury content which is beneficial for heart health, autoimmune diseases, mood disorders, skin, and nails.

All fishes contain omega-3 fatty acids, but some contain them in greater amounts than others. Some of the popular fishes to try out are:

- Salmon.
- Rainbow trout.
- Sardines.
- Mackerel.

A person should eat two average meals of fish that have low mercury content and high omega-3 fatty acids.

GARLIC AND GINGER

"Your body is a bank account, good food choices in it are good investments "

Garlic has been proven to treat and prevent several diseases, while garlic is a primary ingredient for cooking, our ancestors have used it for multiple health purposes. Diallyl disulfide is an anti-inflammatory compound that is found in Garlic that controls the effect of a pro-inflammatory compound known as cytokines.

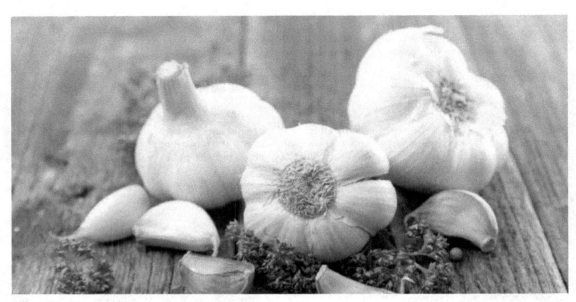

HEALTH BENEFITS OF GARLIC:

- It boosts the immune system.
- It has anti-biotic qualities.
- It improves athletic performance.
- It may prevent Alzheimer's and Dementia.
- It lowers cholesterol.

Ginger has also been known for centuries for its anti-biotic properties not only it has been used for health, it is used for skin care as well for centuries. Ginger has anti-inflammatory properties that promote healthy aging.

HEALTH BENEFITS OF GINGER:

- Improves digestion.
- Mitigate nausea and bad stomach.
- Effective for pain.
- Reduces swelling.

GREEN TEA

Food is the data that quickly alters metabolism, for staying healthy and avoiding obesity metabolism is of prime importance.

Metabolism improves the digestive system which ultimately leads to lower chances of inflammation and that's what green tea can do for the human body. Green tea has been proven to contain anti-oxidants and tea energy-boosting effects.3 cups of green tea daily reduce cancer risk.

Green tea contains EGCG, Aswell - a polyphenol that has anti-inflammatory benefits.

HEALTH BENEFITS OF TEA:

- Improves brain functioning.
- Prevent cardiovascular diseases.
- Prevents bad breath.

HERBS

Herbs don't only smell great but also act great for a healthy body.
- Oregano has amazing anti-oxidant benefits.
- Rosemary and lavender calm anxiety.
- Mint aids in digestion.
- Coriander may slow the growth of cancer cells.

MUSHROOMS

Mushrooms are available worldwide, but not every mushroom is edible. There are only a few edible mushrooms like truffles and portobello mushrooms. Edible mushrooms contain anti-oxidants and in addition to that, they contain vitamin B, copper, and selenium.

Some studies have found that cooking mushrooms can lower their anti-inflammatory properties, so the most preferable way to eat them is raw or slightly cooked.

QUINOA

Quinoa is a gluten-free seed that contains complete protein, a high protein-to-carbohydrate ratio, healthy fats, and fibers. It is both a micro and macronutrient for the human body. It has anti-inflammatory qualities and lowers sugar in the bloodstream and improves heart health.

NOTE:
Always remember to rinse quinoa nicely before using it as it contains a naturally occurring pesticide known as saponin.

TREE NUTS

- Almonds reduce inflammation of blood vessels. They contain vitamin E which is a good source of anti-oxidant.
- Cashews are packed with protein, fiber, and healthy fats. A study demonstrated cashews have anti-inflammatory, anti-oxidative, and analgesic functions.
- Walnut has a high level of omega-3 fatty acids that have been proven to lower LDL.
- Pistachios boost the immune system, keep your heart healthy and provide you with protein and fiber.
- Hazel nuts improve insulin sensitivity, reduce inflammation, and healthy bowel movements.

There are many other anti-inflammatory foods available as well let us enlist some of them too so you never run out of options for a healthy diet,

- Beans.
- Dried chilies.
- Tomatoes.
- Apple.
- Carrots.
- Berries.
- Honey.
- Brocolli.

TOMATOES

Tomatoes are a delicious and nutritious fruit that offer many health benefits. They are a good source of vitamins A and C and are also a good source of lycopene, a powerful antioxidant. Tomatoes have been shown to have anti-inflammatory properties and may help to reduce the risk of some chronic diseases.

KALE
Green leafy vegetables such as kale have a good amount of vitamin E, which is known as a powerful antioxidant that can reduce inflammation.
Some health benefits of kale include:

- Kale may prevent cancer.
- Kale may Improve immunity.
- Kale is beneficial for bone health.

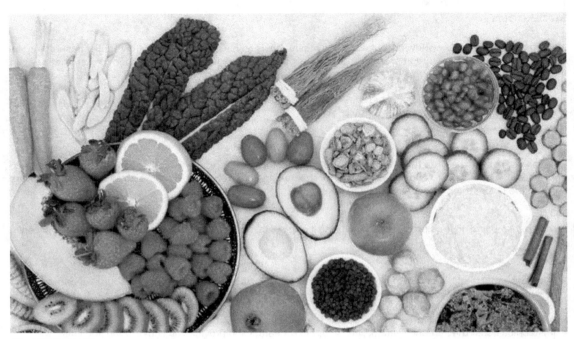

STRAWBERRIES

Scientists have hypothesized that strawberries can prevent colon inflammation by maintaining homeostasis in the colon.

SOME OTHER THE STRAWBERRY HEALTH BENEFITS INCLUDE:

- Strawberries increase good cholesterol.
- Sodium free.
- Strawberries contain low calories.
- strawberries lower blood pressure.
- Prevent cancer.

REFINED SUGAR SUBSTITUTES

You must be thinking if refined sugar is an inflammatory food then what can we use as a sweetener? There are several other options that you can use to sweeten up your food.

STEVIA

Stevia is a plant-based sweetener derived from the leaves of the stevia shrub. Stevia contains no calories but is 450 times sweeter than sugar. Animal research has concluded that stevia can help avoid weight gain and lower blood sugar levels.

DATES

Dates are a great source of fiber, magnesium, vitamin B6, etc. you can use dates in your healthy smoothies as a sugar substitute. Even though dates are high in calories but they do not increase blood sugar levels.

HONEY

Honey is, Golden sweet liquid produced by honeybees that only contains minerals and vitamins but also a good amount of plant compounds that have been found to show great anti-inflammatory properties.

HERBAL REMEDIES

A lot of health workers suggest herbal remedies, such as turmeric to prevent and cure inflammation. According to Dr. Andreew Weil, a natural care specialist says turmeric and ginger are one of the best anti-inflammatory substances. Sadly, Turmeric is not bioavailable as one might think, so you need to combine turmeric with other substances to increase its effects, such as black pepper, coconut oil, etc.

Before You Start Cooking

Before you head into the kitchen right after knowing the anti-inflammatory food let us explain how important planning is. you don't want to have one anti-inflammatory meal and when you head for the next one you either get stuck in the recipe or shortness of food items.

The first thing you need to do is do a weekly meal planning, what you are going to cook throughout the week, and make a breakfast, dinner, lunch, and snack chart. Do check out how long each meal is going to take, time management helps a lot.

The next step is to head out for grocery shopping, all the meals you have listed, note down their ingredients check which one is already available at home and which one is not. Purchase at least a week's worth of groceries.

Budgeting is also really important, as organic food can be sometimes a little expensive, so plan and budget ahead of shopping, and check different market rates as certain stores are more expensive than others.

How to Maintain A Healthy Diet?

You need to eat healthy food as it will help in improving your overall health and also stay fit. But how can you get used to a healthy diet? Here are some tips you can follow:

1. Eat more fruits and vegetables: Fruits are rich in vitamins, minerals, and fibers which are essential for your body. It helps in preventing many diseases such as cancer, heart disease, diabetes, etc. So start eating more fruits to get better results from them.

2. Eat less refined foods: Refined foods lack nutrients like vitamins, minerals, and proteins which are essential for our body. So avoid eating refined foods like white flour products, white sugar, etc., which are not good for our health since they contain little nutrients or hardly any nutrients at all.

3. Studies have also found that lifestyle adoptions can also turn out to be quite effective against chronic inflammation. This includes stress reduction techniques such as yoga, meditation, exercise, etc.

WRAPPING UP THE HEALTHY TORTILLA

First, if we haven't lost you yet, I'd like to take a moment to say thank you for reading this article. There's no greater joy than sharing information with people who are interested in it – it's why I write. And if you're still here, I'm happy to tell you that inflammation is one of the worst things that can happen to our bodies. While it is important in fighting off infection and healing wounds, chronic inflammation is a key factor in many of the most devastating diseases of our time. A healthy diet can help curb some of the symptoms of chronic inflammation and has been shown to reduce its effects.

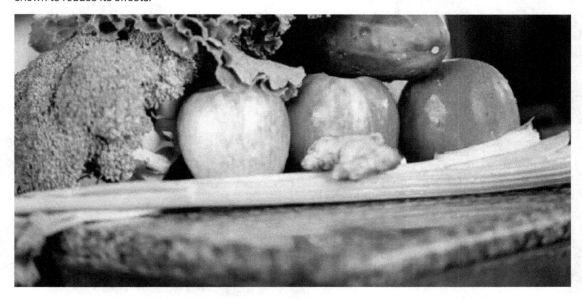

Chapter 3
28-Day Whole Foods Meal Plan Challenge

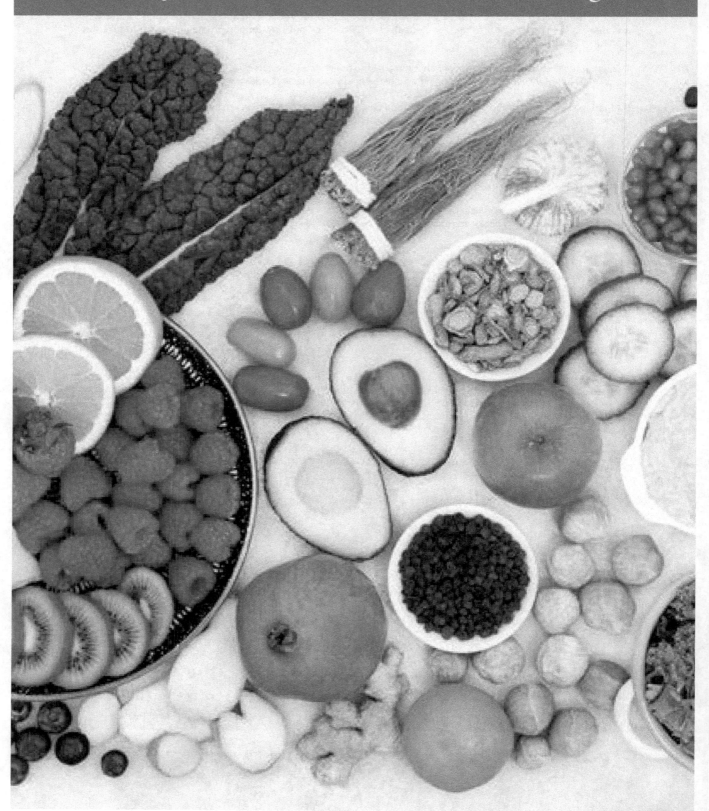

Meal Plan	Breakfast	Lunch	Dinner	Motivational Quotes
Day-1	Turmeric Lassi	Chicken Satay	Herb Omelet	It makes no difference how slowly you move as long as you don't stop.

Proper Scheduling

Adhering to a restricted diet requires meticulous preparation and timing. Whenever works best for you is when you should start eating a diet based solely on whole foods. Make it work for your schedule. Events in your life, both planned and unplanned, can throw off your meal plan. If you want to stick to your diet and not give up halfway through, it's important to pick a time of year that is conducive to your lifestyle.

Meal Plan	Breakfast	Lunch	Dinner	Motivational Quotes
Day-2	Turmeric Lassi	Picante Trout Fillets	Vegetable Curry	Don't let a mishap in the road put an end to your journey.

Control is essential, but following through on your plans is even better.

No challenge, not even a 28-day challenge of eating only whole foods, can be completed without careful preparation. If you do your planning right, you shouldn't have to worry about anything throwing a wrench into your plans. You need to be organized and well-prepared at all times if you want to succeed with this diet. You should bring a whole meals compliant lunch if you have to eat at your desk. If you find yourself in a situation where you must eat away from home, it is important to take the time to research the menu items to ensure that you can stay on track with your whole meals challenge.

Meal Plan	Breakfast	Lunch	Dinner	Motivational Quotes
Day-3	Cider Spritzer	Tofu Cabbage Stir-Fry	Spanish Rice	Don't dig your own grave with your own knife and fork.

Examine Nutrition Labels Thoroughly

It's important to remember that non-compliant ingredients, such as those used in processing, can hide in foods like processed meat, so it's best to check the labels before eating anything. Also, many of your favorite foods, like ham, have added sugars. You can only succeed in this challenge if you keep a close eye on what you eat and always read the labels. If you're unsure about whether or not to consume an ingredient, you can learn more about it by conducting a simple online search.

Meal Plan	Breakfast	Lunch	Dinner	Motivational Quotes
Day-4	Santa Barbara Migas	Ginger Fruit Salad	Lime Lentil Soup	You feel crap when you eat crap. Continue your journey.

You should take a break every now and again.

You can save money and time in the kitchen by following this 28-day meal plan. Spending more money on pre-prepared time-saving ingredients is preferable to spending more time in the kitchen. It will be well worth it in the long run.

Meal Plan	Breakfast	Lunch	Dinner	Motivational Quotes
Day-5	Turkey-Maple Breakfast Sausages	Parsnip & Tilapia Bake	Cilantro Okra	Take things slowly at first.

So much Dishes to Discover

Your diet plan has been extended by 28 days. Prepare some of your most daring culinary creations yet. This means no more boring meals or routine preparations. There'll be more to it than just eating right for a month and a half. It will also be a time of discovery, merriment, and exciting new experiences. If you're lucky, you'll find a few go-to recipes that you can use again and again during this time.

Day-6	Allergen-Free Breakfast Cookies	Mushroom Lettuce Wraps	Italian Bean Soup	When you want to give up, remember why you started.

Twenty-Eight days may go rather quickly.

Your 28-day whole foods challenge will tire you out, as will anything else. But if you keep going and don't give up. The month of February will fly by faster than you think. Never forget that success rarely comes easily. Furthermore, if you follow the plan for the full 28 days. When you look back, you'll be pleased with yourself.

Day-7	Chia-Cherry Oats	Persian Saucy Sole	Basic Beans	When, if not now?

It is not a smart idea to binge.

You shouldn't go crazy on the food and the portions just because you're about to start a diet. This is a terrible plan 99 times out of 100. Even though this is not a diet, the first few days of the 28-day challenge may make you feel hungry and tempted to binge. Try to refrain from doing that.

Day-8	Banana Oat Pancakes	Gingered Broccoli Soup	Mushroom Pizza	Fall seven times, rise eight times.

When dining out, place your order as soon as possible.

It's best to place your order as soon as possible while perusing a restaurant's menu and then put the menu down. When you spend a considerable amount of time deliberating over your order and perusing the menu. A non-compliant item on the menu could easily derail your 28-day diet plan. Being fully invested in this course is essential. It's a wise financial move.

Day-9	Orange-Glazed Raspberry Muffins	Chard Trout Fillets	Citrus Asparagus	Every step, no matter how small, is a step in the right direction.

Freeze a couple meals

Stocking your freezer need not be a source of stress, but having a few things that can be used quickly is helpful for days when you come home from work exhausted and need to make food quickly. Despite your hunger, you won't feel like eating anything. Consequently, if you find yourself with some spare time on your hands, it is wise to cook up some meals and put them away in the freezer. You're going to want to have some.

Day-10	Breakfast "Fried Rice"	Rosemary Pork Loin	Yummy Fish Curry	Taking it one pound at a time.

Remove any junk food from your diet.

The presence of junk food in the home increases the likelihood that its inhabitants will succumb to the urge to eat it. Temptation should not be met head-on, as there is no need to test your resolve. You should get rid of all the junk food in your house before starting this 28-day meal plan. You'll be free from distractions and better able to focus on your goals if you do this.

Day-11	Sweet Orange Crepes	Fish Stew	Basil Beet Pasta	You'll wish you'd started today a year from now.

Stay away from enticing situations.

The elimination of junk food is just the beginning. It's also important to stay away from anything that might tempt you. You should always be aware of your immediate environment, decline restaurant invitations with caution, and keep your wits about you to avoid becoming a victim of distraction. Don't put the whole program at risk like that.

Day-12	Sweet Orange Crepes	Korean-Style Buckwheat	Coconut & Tofu Soup	With each new day comes new strength and new ideas.

Make Plans for Your Life Outside of work

While taking the Whole Foods 28-Day Challenge, it is not necessary to isolate yourself from friends and family. You shouldn't shut yourself away from the world, but you also shouldn't let your program's integrity be compromised by letting your guard down.

Day-13	Coconut Oat Bread	Chocolate Chili	Turkey-Pecan Salad	Stop slacking and start making things happen.

Avoid deceptive and phony treats.

Some people believe that making treats or desserts with whole foods complaint ingredients is acceptable. However, the opposite is true. Do not do anything. You must be disciplined in order to stay on track. There is no need for compromise.

Day-14	Simple Apple Muffins	Greek-Style Sea Bass	Sunday Pork Tacos	The past is unchangeable, but the future is still within your grasp.

Overeating Foods Should Be Avoided

Certain foods can set off a binge-eating episode. You must accept responsibility for identifying these trigger foods and attempting to avoid them as much as possible.

Day-15	Chocolate-Mango Quinoa Bowl	Baked Basil Chicken	Coconut Fruit Salad	Failure does not exist: you either win or learn.

Start making Leftover food Your BFF

The preparation of meals will be a lot less of a hassle if you make double the amount of food. You'll spend less time cooking thanks to leftovers, and you won't have to worry as much about what to eat every day.

Day-16	Lemony Quinoa Muffins	Sicilian Chicken Bake	Garlic Veggie Bisque	You can never win if you never start.

Shop for Long-Lasting Ingredients That Aren't Expensive

Eating healthy is not cheap; in fact, it is quite costly. As a result, starting and sticking to this meal plan requires a lot of willpower. When shopping, choose items that will last you a long time so you don't have to keep spending. Even if you're on a tight budget, this should come in handy.

Day-17	Morning Pecan & Pear Farro	Minty Eggplant Salad	Sardine Donburi	You are your only constraint.

Keep your scale at a safe distance from your body.

You will be tempted to continue weighing yourself while on this diet, especially if you are several days into your challenge and want to know what has happened to your weight. To avoid this temptation, keep your weighing scale out of sight.

Day-18	Blueberry Muesli Breakfast	Thyme Pork Loin Bake	Picante Trout Fillets	Success is not an accident: it is the result of hard work and perseverance.

Weight loss should not be the primary goal.

If you want to lose weight, that's great, but your main goal in this meal plan should be to lose weight. Don't begin the program with the sole goal of losing weight; instead, focus on healthy eating first, with weight loss coming in a close second.

Day-19	Turkey-Maple Breakfast Sausages	Olive & Salmon Quinoa	Bulgur & Kale Salad	You will reap the benefits of what you plant now.

Physical activity is essential.

The simple act of walking around can improve our mood. The result is less anxiety and a better disposition. No matter what kind of exercise you do, you'll reap the health benefits. Morning strolls, jogs, and runs are all great ways to start the day off on the path to better health.

Day-20	Simple Apple Muffins	Ginger Squash Soup	Herby Green Whole Chicken	If you know you can do better, then go ahead and do it.

It is critical to maintain a positive attitude.

It is critical that you set yourself up for success as you embark on this journey, and this begins with your mind. It's all about having a positive mindset. You might not be able to achieve anything you can't imagine. You will succeed if you believe you will.

Day-21	Almond Oatmeal Porridge	Baked Cod Fillets with Mushroom	Tamari Tofu with Sweet Potatoes & Broccoli	Never let your fears dictate your destiny.

Herbal Teas are beneficial.

Herbal teas are great because they allow you to try new flavors without jeopardizing your diet. If you get a craving for something sweet, you can sip on a herbal tea of your choice. You will not jeopardize your meal plan, and you will eat healthily. It is a win-win situation.

Day-22	Pecan & Pumpkin Seed Oat Jars	Mumbai-Inspired Chicken	Green Pasta Salad	It is never too late to make amends.

Soups

Instead of drinking sugary drinks, try replacing them with delicious and healthy soups. Soups allow you to experiment with different flavors. You can make a large number of them. Make them nutritious, tasty, and inexpensive.

| Day-23 | Santa Barbara Migas | Pomodoro Cream Soup | White Pizza with Mixed Mushrooms | The net will appear if you leap. |

Simplicity

It is usually best to keep things simple. Overachievement can lead to disappointment. So, each week, try a new recipe, but keep things simple. It will make the program easier for you to understand.

| Day-24 | Spinach & Leek Frittata | Apple-Ginger Pork Chops | Easy Garbanzo Soup | The key to change is to devote all of your energy to building the new rather than fighting the old. |

Always keep an emergency supply of food on hand.

You may become hungry at inconvenient times. Having emergency meals on hand can be extremely beneficial. Make simple foods and keep them on hand for when you need them.

| Day-25 | Coconut Oat Bread | Smoky Lamb Souvlaki | Thai Sweet Potato Soup | You get what you concentrate on, so concentrate on what you want. |

Your go-to foods include:

It's always a good idea to identify your go-to foods and keep them close at hand. When you do this, you'll be able to quickly prepare meals when you're hungry. Fruits can also be used as substitutes for sweets if you are craving something sweet.

| Day-26 | Breakfast "Fried Rice" | Jerk Chicken Drumsticks | Coconutty Brown Rice | Yes, I believe I can. |

Increase your protein intake by twofold.

Most whole-food eaters don't get enough protein. A 2,000-calorie diet should have at least 100 grams of protein. 4-6oz of eggs, fish, red meat, or poultry every meal. Animal protein is full and easy to absorb. (Don't confuse protein grams with meat weight.)

| Day-27 | Chia-Cherry Oats | Veggie "Fried" Quinoa | Chickpea and Kale Salad | Don't give up until you're satisfied. |

Don't eat too many Fruits.

Fruits are delicious, but replacing sweets and candy with multiple servings of fruits will not help you break your sugar addiction. As a result, limit your fruit intake to one or two servings per day.

| Day-28 | Spinach & Leek Frittata | Za`atar Pork Tenderloin | Noodle Soup | A small amount of progress each day adds up to big results. |

Your Meals Shouldn't Be Drunk

Smoothies are technically permitted, but it is important to remember that consuming too many calories is not a good idea. So, do yourself a favor and cut down on the number of drinkable meals and calories you consume each day.

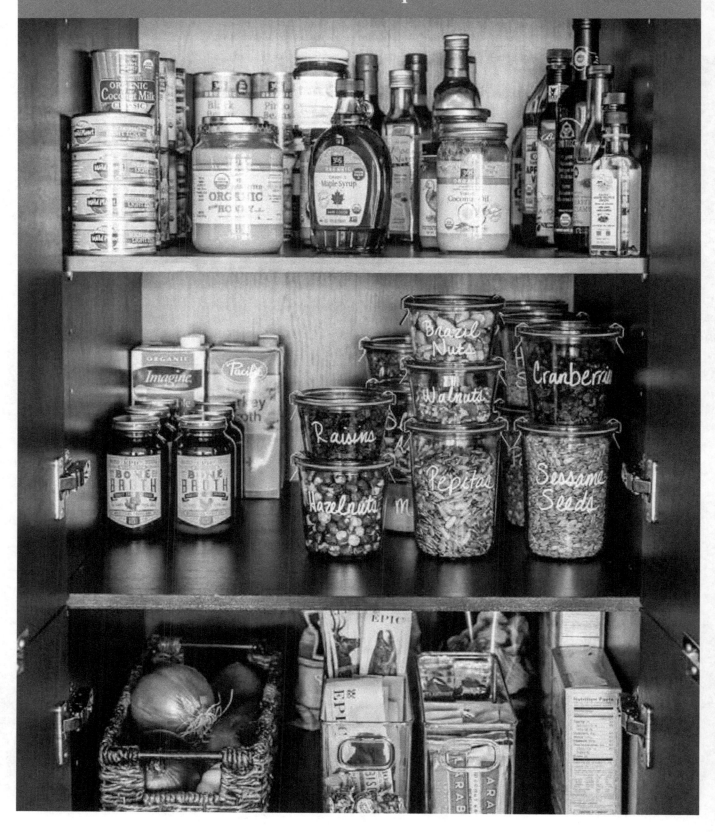

Chapter 4
Kitchen Staples

Beans

Prep time: 5 minutes, plus overnight soaking time | Cook time: 1 hour| Makes 2½ cups cooked beans

- 8 ounces dried beans
- Filtered water, for soaking and cooking
- Pinch salt
- Seasonings, such as bay leaves, garlic, onion, cumin (optional)

1. In a large glass bowl, cover the beans with water. Add the salt and let soak on the counter, covered, overnight.
2. Drain the beans and rinse well. Transfer to a large pot and add any seasonings you like (if using).
3. Cover the beans with 1 to 2 inches of water, place the pot over high heat, and bring to a boil. Reduce heat to low and simmer for 1 hour.
4. Check the beans for doneness; some varieties require longer cooking times. Continue to simmer, if needed, and check every 10 minutes until done. Use immediately in soups or chilis, or refrigerate in an airtight container for up to 1 week. Cooked beans can also be frozen for up to 3 months.

PER SERVING(½ CUP)

Calories: 153; Total Fat: 1g; Saturated Fat: 0g; Cholesterol: 0mg; Carbohydrates: 28g; Fiber: 7g; Protein: 10g

Almond-Hazelnut Milk

Prep time: 15 minutes| Makes about 4 cups

- ½ cup soaked raw hazelnuts, drained (See Preparation Tip)
- ½ cup soaked raw almonds, drained (See Preparation Tip)
- 4 cups filtered water
- 1 teaspoon raw honey (optional)
- ¼ teaspoon vanilla extract (optional)

1. In a colander, combine the hazelnuts and almonds and give them a good rinse. Transfer to a blender and add the water. Blend at high speed for 30 seconds.
2. Place a nut milk bag (see Equipment Tip) or other meshlike material over a large bowl and carefully pour the nut mixture into it.
3. Pick up the top of the bag and strain the liquid into the bowl, squeezing the pulp to remove as much liquid as possible.
4. Using a funnel, transfer the nut milk to a sealable bottle. Add the honey (if using) and vanilla (if using). Seal the bottle and shake well. Refrigerate for up to 4 days.
5. The raw nuts can be soaked together, for at least seven hours, with 1 tablespoon of sea salt (this will get rinsed off so it doesn't affect sodium levels).

PER SERVING(1 CUP)

Calories: 85; Total Fat: 5g; Saturated Fat: 0g; Cholesterol: 0mg; Carbohydrates: 10g; Fiber: 1g; Protein: 2g

Lemon Dijon Mustard Dressing

Prep time: 5 minutes| Makes about 6 tablespoons

- ¼ cup extra-virgin olive oil
- 2 tablespoons freshly squeezed lemon juice
- 1 teaspoon Dijon mustard
- ½ teaspoon raw honey
- 1 garlic clove, minced
- ¼ teaspoon dried basil
- ¼ teaspoon salt

1. In a glass jar with a lid, combine the olive oil, lemon juice, mustard, honey, garlic, basil, and salt.
2. Cover and shake vigorously until the ingredients are well combined and emulsified. Refrigerate for up to 1 week.

PER SERVING(1½ TABLESPOONS)

Calories: 128; Total Fat: 13.5g; Saturated Fat: 1.8g; Cholesterol: 0mg; Carbohydrates: 1.8g; Fiber: 0.1g; Protein: 0.1g

Tahini-Lime Dressing

Prep time: 5 minutes| Makes about ¾ cup

- ⅓ cup tahini (sesame paste)
- 3 tablespoons filtered water
- 2 tablespoons freshly squeezed lime juice
- 1 tablespoon apple cider vinegar
- 1 teaspoon lime zest
- 1½ teaspoons raw honey
- ¼ teaspoon garlic powder
- ¼ teaspoon salt

1. In a glass jar with a lid, combine the tahini, water, lime juice, vinegar, lime zest, honey, garlic powder, and salt.
2. Cover and shake vigorously until the ingredients are well combined and emulsified. Refrigerate for up to 1 week.

PER SERVING(1½ TABLESPOONS)

Calories: 157; Total Fat: 12.6g; Saturated Fat: 2.1g; Cholesterol: 0mg; Carbohydrates: 5.1g; Fiber: 0g; Protein: 6.2g

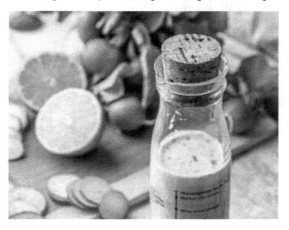

Paleo Caesar Dressing

Prep time: 10 minutes| Makes about ½ cup

- ¼ cup Paleo mayonnaise
- 2 tablespoons extra-virgin olive oil
- 2 tablespoons freshly squeezed lemon juice
- ½ teaspoon lemon zest
- 2 garlic cloves, minced
- 1 tablespoon white wine vinegar
- ½ teaspoon anchovy paste
- ¼ teaspoon salt
- Freshly ground black pepper

1. In a small bowl, whisk the mayonnaise, olive oil, lemon juice, lemon zest, garlic, vinegar, anchovy paste, and salt until well combined and emulsified.
2. Season with pepper. Cover and refrigerate for up to 1 week.

PER SERVING(2 TABLESPOONS)

Calories: 167; Total Fat: 18.9g; Saturated Fat: 2.4g; Cholesterol: 22.3mg; Carbohydrates: 1.3g; Fiber: 0.3g; Protein: 0.2g

The Everything Aioli

Prep time: 5 minutes| Makes about ½ cup

- ½ cup plain whole-milk yogurt
- 2 teaspoons Dijon mustard
- ½ teaspoon hot sauce
- ¼ teaspoon raw honey
- Pinch salt

1. In a small bowl, stir together the yogurt, mustard, hot sauce, honey, and salt. Serve immediately, or cover and refrigerate for up to 3 days.

PER SERVING(2 TABLESPOONS)

Calories: 43; Total Fat: 2.4g; Saturated Fat: 1.5g; Cholesterol: 10mg; Carbohydrates: 3.2g; Fiber: 0g; Protein: 2g

Pistachio Pesto

Prep time: 10 minutes| Makes 4 cups

- 2 cups tightly packed fresh basil leaves
- 1 cup raw pistachios
- ½ cup extra-virgin olive oil, divided
- ½ cup shredded raw Parmesan cheese
- 2 teaspoons freshly squeezed lemon juice
- ½ teaspoon garlic powder
- ¼ teaspoon salt
- Freshly ground black pepper

1. In a food processor (or blender), combine the basil, pistachios, and ¼ cup of olive oil. Blend for 15 seconds.
2. Add the cheese, lemon juice, garlic powder, and salt, and season with pepper.
3. With the processor running, slowly pour in the remaining ¼ cup of olive oil until all ingredients are well combined. Serve immediately, cover and refrigerate for up to 5 days, or freeze for 3 to 4 months.

PER SERVING(4 OUNCES)

Calories: 229; Total Fat: 22.3g; Saturated Fat: 3.6g; Cholesterol: 4.8mg; Carbohydrates: 3.8g; Fiber: 1.7g; Protein: 5.5g

Almond Romesco Sauce

Prep time: 10 minutes | Cook time: 10 minutes| Makes 2 cups

- 2 red bell peppers, roughly chopped
- 5 or 6 cherry tomatoes, roughly chopped
- 3 garlic cloves, roughly chopped
- ½ white onion, roughly chopped
- 1 tablespoon avocado oil
- 1 cup blanched raw almonds
- ¼ cup extra-virgin olive oil
- 2 tablespoons apple cider vinegar
- ¼ teaspoon salt
- Freshly ground black pepper

1. Preheat the broiler to high.
2. Line a baking sheet with aluminum foil. Spread the bell peppers, tomatoes, garlic, and onion on the prepared sheet and drizzle with the avocado oil. Broil for 10 minutes.
3. In a food processor (or blender), pulse the almonds until they resemble bread crumbs.
4. Add the broiled vegetables, olive oil, vinegar, and salt, and season with pepper. Process until smooth. Serve immediately. Cover and refrigerate for up to 5 days, or freeze for 3 to 4 months.

PER SERVING(4 OUNCES)

Calories: 358; Total Fat: 32.2g; Saturated Fat: 3.2g; Cholesterol: 0mg; Carbohydrates: 13.7g; Fiber: 6.4g; Protein: 7.3g

Mild Curry Powder

Prep time: 5 minutes | Cook time: 5 minutes| Makes ¼ cup

- 1 tablespoon ground turmeric
- 1 tablespoon ground cumin
- 2 teaspoons ground coriander
- 1 teaspoon ground cardamom
- 1 teaspoon ground cinnamon
- 1 teaspoon ground ginger
- ½ teaspoon fenugreek powder
- ½ teaspoon ground cloves

1. In a small bowl, stir together the turmeric, cumin, coriander, cardamom, cinnamon, ginger, fenugreek, and cloves until well blended.
2. Store the curry powder in an airtight container for up to 1 month.

PER SERVING(1 TEASPOON)

Calories: 6; Total fat: 0g; Saturated fat: 0g; Carbohydrates: 1g; Fiber: 0g; Protein: 0g

Mediterranean Rub

Prep time: 5 minutes | Cook time: 5 minutes| Makes ¾ cup

- ¼ cup packed coconut sugar
- 3 tablespoons dried oregano leaves
- 2 tablespoons dried thyme leaves
- 1 tablespoon dried tarragon
- 1 teaspoon dried marjoram
- 1 teaspoon dried dill
- 1 teaspoon dried basil

1. In a small bowl, stir together the coconut sugar, oregano, thyme, tarragon, marjoram, dill, and basil until well blended.
2. Store the seasoning in a sealed container for up to 1 month.

PER SERVING(1 TEASPOON)

Calories: 5; Total fat: 0g; Saturated fat: 0g; Carbohydrates: 1g; Fiber: 0g; Protein: 0g

Spicy Tunisian Vinaigrette

Prep time: 5 minutes | Cook time: 5 minutes| Makes 1¼ cup

- ¾ cup olive oil
- ¼ cup apple cider vinegar
- 1 tablespoon freshly squeezed lemon juice
- ¼ cup chopped fresh parsley
- 1 teaspoon bottled minced garlic
- 1 teaspoon ground cumin
- ¼ teaspoon ground coriander
- Pinch sea salt

1. In a medium bowl, whisk the olive oil, cider vinegar, and lemon juice until emulsified.
2. Whisk in the parsley, garlic, cumin, and coriander.
3. Season with sea salt.
4. Refrigerate the vinaigrette in a sealed container for up to 2 weeks.

PER SERVING(2 TABLESPOONS)

Calories: 133; Total fat: 15g; Saturated fat: 2g; Carbohydrates: 0g; Fiber: 0g; Protein: 0g

Traditional Gremolata Sauce

Prep time: 5 minutes | Cook time: 10 minutes| Makes 1 cup

- ¾ cup finely chopped fresh parsley
- Juice of 2 lemons (or 6 tablespoons)
- Zest of 2 lemons (optional)
- 2 tablespoons olive oil
- 2 teaspoons bottled minced garlic
- ¼ teaspoon sea salt

1. In a small bowl, stir together the parsley, lemon juice, lemon zest (if using), olive oil, garlic, and sea salt until well blended.
2. Refrigerate in a sealed container for up to 4 days.

PER SERVING(2 TABLESPOONS)

Calories: 33; Total fat: 4g; Saturated fat: 1g; Carbohydrates: 1g; Fiber: 0g; Protein: 0g

Creamy Sesame Dressing

Prep time: 5 minutes | Cook time: 5 minutes| Makes ¾ cup

- ½ cup canned full-fat coconut milk
- 2 tablespoons tahini
- 2 tablespoons freshly squeezed lime juice
- 1 teaspoon bottled minced garlic
- 1 teaspoon minced fresh chives
- Pinch sea salt

1. In a small bowl, whisk the coconut milk, tahini, lime juice, garlic, and chives until well blended. You can also prepare this in a blender.
2. Season with sea salt and transfer the dressing to a container with a lid. Refrigerate for up to 1 week.

PER SERVING(1 TABLESPOON)

Calories: 40; Total fat: 4g; Saturated fat: 2g; Carbohydrates: 2g; Fiber: 0g; Protein: 1g

Maple Dressing

Prep time: 5 minutes | Cook time: 5 minutes| Makes 1¼ cup

- 1 cup canned full-fat coconut milk
- 2 tablespoons pure maple syrup
- 1 tablespoon Dijon mustard
- 1 tablespoon apple cider vinegar
- Sea salt

1. In a medium bowl, whisk the coconut milk, maple syrup, mustard, and cider vinegar until smoothly blended. Season with sea salt. You can also prepare this in a blender.
2. Refrigerate the dressing in a sealed container for up to 1 week.

PER SERVING(2 TABLESPOONS)

Calories: 67; Total fat: 6g; Saturated fat: 5g; Carbohydrates: 4g; Fiber: 1g; Protein: 1g

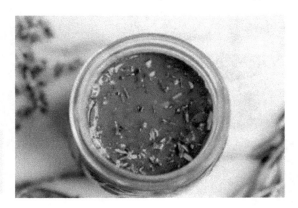

Avocado-Herb Spread

Prep time: 5 minutes | Cook time: 5 minutes | Makes 1 cup

- 1 avocado, peeled and pitted
- 2 tablespoons freshly squeezed lemon juice
- 2 tablespoons chopped fresh parsley
- 1 teaspoon chopped fresh dill
- ½ teaspoon ground coriander
- Sea salt
- Freshly ground black pepper

1. In a blender, pulse the avocado until smoothly puréed.
2. Add the lemon juice, parsley, dill, and coriander. Pulse until well blended.
3. Season with sea salt and pepper.
4. Refrigerate the spread in a sealed container for up to 4 days.

PER SERVING(2 TABLESPOONS)

Calories: 53; Total fat: 5g; Saturated fat: 1g; Carbohydrates: 2g; Fiber: 2g; Protein: 1g

Peach Butter

Prep time: 5 minutes | Cook time: 3 hours, 30 minutes | Makes 2 cups

- 8 peaches (about 3 pounds), peeled, pitted, and chopped, or about 6 cups frozen, sliced peaches
- Water, for cooking
- ¼ cup raw honey

1. In a large saucepan over high heat, combine the peaches with enough water to cover the fruit by about 1 inch. Bring the liquid to a boil.
2. Reduce the heat to low and simmer for about 3 hours, stirring frequently until the mixture resembles a thick applesauce.
3. Stir in the honey. Simmer for about 30 minutes until the mixture starts to caramelize. Remove the peach butter from the heat and let it cool for 30 minutes.
4. Spoon the mixture into a container and cool completely before covering. Keep refrigerated for up to 2 weeks.

PER SERVING(2 TABLESPOONS)

Calories: 46; Total fat: 0g; Saturated fat: 0g; Carbohydrates: 11g; Fiber: 1g; Protein: 1g

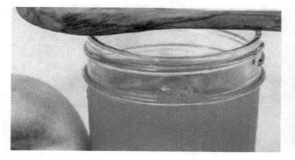

Sweet Carrot Spread

Prep time: 5 minutes | Cook time: 10 minutes | Makes 2 cups

- 3 carrots, peeled and cut into chunks
- ½ cup almonds
- 2 tablespoons freshly squeezed lemon juice
- 1 tablespoon pure maple syrup
- ½ teaspoon ground cardamom
- Sea salt

1. In a food processor, pulse the carrots until very finely chopped.
2. Add the almonds, lemon juice, maple syrup, and cardamom. Process until smooth.
3. Season the spread with sea salt and transfer to a lidded container. Refrigerate for up to 6 days.

PER SERVING(2 TABLESPOONS)

Calories: 26; Total fat: 2g; Saturated fat: 0g; Carbohydrates: 3g; Fiber: 1g; Protein: 1g

Parsley Chimichurri

Prep time: 5 minutes | Cook time: 10 minutes | Makes 1 cup

- 1 cup coarsely chopped fresh parsley
- ½ cup fresh mint leaves
- ¼ cup olive oil
- 2 tablespoons freshly squeezed lemon juice
- 2 teaspoons bottled minced garlic
- Pinch sea salt

1. In a blender or food processor, combine the parsley, mint, olive oil, lemon juice, garlic, and sea salt. Pulse until the herbs are very finely chopped and the ingredients are well mixed.
2. Refrigerate the mixture in a sealed container for up to 1 week.

PER SERVING(2 TABLESPOONS)

Calories: 61; Total fat: 6g; Saturated fat: 1g; Carbohydrates: 1g; Fiber: 1g; Protein: 1g

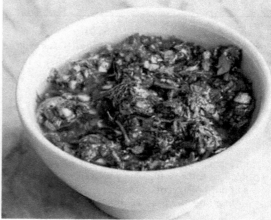

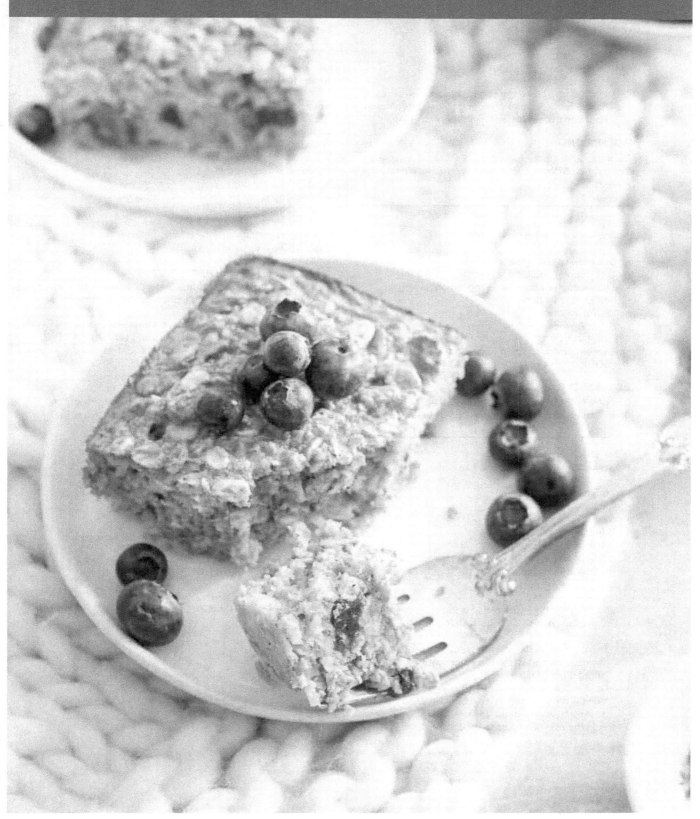

Turmeric Lassi

Prep time: 5 minutes| Serves 2

- 2 cups plain whole-milk yogurt, or milk kefir
- 1 banana
- 1 tablespoon freshly squeezed lemon juice
- 2 teaspoons raw honey
- 1 teaspoon ground turmeric
- ½ teaspoon ground cinnamon
- ¼ teaspoon ground ginger

1. In a blender, blend the yogurt, banana, lemon juice, honey, turmeric, cinnamon, and ginger until smooth. Pour into two tall glasses and serve immediately.

PER SERVING

Calories: 234; Total Fat: 8.2g; Saturated Fat: 5.2g; Cholesterol: 31.9mg; Carbohydrates: 33.5g; Fiber: 2.2g; Protein: 9.3g

Cider Spritzer

Prep time: 5 minutes| Serves 1

- 8 ounces sparkling water
- 1 tablespoon apple cider vinegar
- 1 tablespoon freshly squeezed lemon juice
- Few drops raw honey
- Ice, for serving

1. In a tall glass, gently stir together the sparkling water, vinegar, lemon juice, and honey. Pour over ice and serve immediately.

PER SERVING

Calories: 6; Total Fat: 0g; Saturated Fat: 0g; Cholesterol: 0mg; Carbohydrates: 1.8g; Fiber: 0g; Protein: 0.1g

Santa Barbara Migas

Prep time: 10 minutes | Cook time: 10 minutes| Serves 4

- 1 tablespoon avocado oil
- ½ onion, diced
- 8 eggs
- ¾ teaspoon salt
- ½ teaspoon garlic powder
- ½ teaspoon freshly ground black pepper
- ½ cup plantain chips, crushed
- ½ cup salsa
- 2 avocados, sliced
- Splash of freshly squeezed lime juice
- Fresh cilantro leaves, for garnish (optional)

1. In a small skillet over medium heat, add the avocado oil and sauté the onion until translucent, about 5 minutes
2. In a medium bowl, whisk the eggs, salt, garlic powder, and pepper. Add to the skillet, and stir until cooked to your desired doneness, 2 to 3 minutes.
3. Add the plantain chips to the egg mixture. Stir well

and remove the skillet from the heat.
4. Top with the salsa and avocado. Sprinkle with the lime juice. Garnish with cilantro (if using) and serve immediately.

PER SERVING

Calories: 374; Total Fat: 27g; Saturated Fat: 6g; Cholesterol: 370mg; Carbohydrates: 22g; Fiber: 6g; Protein: 14g

Granola Cups with Yogurt

Prep time: 10 minutes | Cook time: 10 minutes| Serves 4

- 1 cup rolled oats
- ½ cup almond flour
- 2 tablespoons coconut sugar
- ½ teaspoon baking soda
- ½ cup dried cranberries, blueberries, or goji berries
- ¼ cup pecans, chopped
- ¼ cup sliced almonds
- 2 tablespoons unsweetened dried coconut
- 4 tablespoons coconut oil, divided
- 3 tablespoons pure maple syrup
- 1 teaspoon vanilla extract
- 2 cups plain whole-milk yogurt

1. Preheat the oven to 325°F.
2. In a medium bowl, mix the oats, almond flour, coconut sugar, baking soda, dried berries, pecans, almonds, and coconut.
3. In a microwave-safe bowl, melt 3 tablespoons of coconut oil. Stir in the maple syrup and vanilla. Add the coconut oil-maple syrup to the oat mixture and stir well to combine.
4. Using the remaining 1 tablespoon of coconut oil, lightly coat the cups of a standard muffin tin.
5. Evenly divide the granola mixture among the cups, pressing it in to create a bowl shape in each cup. Bake for 10 minutes. Cool completely before carefully removing the cups.
6. Fill each cup with some of the yogurt and serve.

PER SERVING

Calories: 183; Total Fat: 12g; Saturated Fat: 6g; Cholesterol: 5mg; Carbohydrates: 12g; Fiber: 3g; Protein: 4g

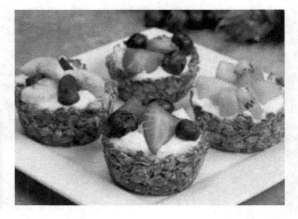

Spinach & Leek Frittata

Prep time: 5 minutes | Cook time: 20 minutes| Serves 4

- 2 leeks (white and pale green parts only), thoroughly washed and finely chopped
- 2 tablespoons avocado oil
- 8 eggs
- ¾ teaspoon salt
- ½ teaspoon garlic powder
- ½ teaspoon dried basil
- 1 cup packed fresh baby spinach leaves, thoroughly washed and dried
- 1 cup sliced cremini mushrooms
- Freshly ground black pepper

1. Preheat the oven to 400°F.
2. In a large ovenproof skillet over medium-high heat, sauté the leeks in the avocado oil for about 5 minutes until soft.
3. In a medium bowl, whisk the eggs, salt, garlic powder, and basil. Add to the skillet with the leeks. Cook for 5 minutes, stirring frequently.
4. Stir in the spinach and mushrooms. Season with pepper. Transfer the skillet to the oven. Bake for 10 minutes, or until the eggs are firmly set.

PER SERVING

Calories: 276; Total Fat: 17g; Saturated Fat: 4g; Cholesterol: 372mg; Carbohydrates: 15g; Fiber: 3g; Protein: 19g

Breakfast "Fried Rice"

Prep time: 10 minutes | Cook time: 15 minutes| Serves 2

- ½ white onion, diced
- 2 garlic cloves, minced
- 1 tablespoon avocado oil
- ¼ cup non-GMO organic sweet corn kernels
- ¼ cup peas
- ¼ cup shredded carrots
- 2 cups cooked rice
- 1 tablespoon sesame oil
- 2 eggs, whisked
- Dash red pepper flakes
- ¼ teaspoon salt
- Freshly ground black pepper

1. In a medium skillet over medium heat, sauté the onion and garlic in the avocado oil until translucent, about 5 minutes.
2. Add the rice and sesame oil, breaking the rice up with a spoon. As the rice begins to soften, add the eggs. Cook, stirring occasionally, until thoroughly cooked, about 5 minutes.
3. Sprinkle with the red pepper flakes and salt, and season with pepper. Serve immediately.

PER SERVING

Calories: 453; Total Fat: 19g; Saturated Fat: 43; Cholesterol: 186mg; Carbohydrates: 59g; Fiber: 3g; Protein: 13g

Allergen-Free Breakfast Cookies

Prep time: 10 minutes | Cook time: 12 minutes| Makes 10 cookies

- 3 very ripe bananas
- ½ cup almond butter
- 2 tablespoons raw honey
- 1 tablespoon coconut oil, melted
- 2 teaspoons vanilla extract
- 1 teaspoon baking powder
- 1 teaspoon ground cinnamon
- ½ teaspoon salt
- 2½ cups rolled oats

1. Preheat the oven to 350°F.
2. Line a large baking sheet with parchment paper.
3. In a large bowl, mash the bananas with a potato masher or a fork.
4. Stir in the almond butter, honey, coconut oil, and vanilla until well mixed.
5. Sprinkle in the baking powder, cinnamon, and salt. Add the oats and chocolate chips (if using) in batches, stirring after each addition until all ingredients are incorporated.
6. Place heaping tablespoons of dough onto the prepared sheet, leaving at least 1 inch between dough balls. Bake for 10 to 12 minutes.
7. Let the cookies rest in the pan for 5 minutes, and then transfer to a cooling rack. These cookies will keep refrigerated in a sealed container for several days.

PER SERVING

Calories: 306; Total Fat: 16g; Saturated Fat: 5g; Cholesterol: 0mg; Carbohydrates: 39g; Fiber: 5g; Protein: 7g

Turkey-Maple Breakfast Sausages

Prep time: 10 minutes | Cook time: 12 minutes| Makes 8 sausages

- 1 pound ground turkey
- 1½ tablespoons pure maple syrup
- 1 teaspoon salt
- ½ teaspoon freshly ground black pepper
- ½ teaspoon garlic powder
- ½ teaspoon dried oregano
- ¼ teaspoon red pepper flakes
- 2 tablespoons ghee

1. In a large bowl, mix the turkey, maple syrup, salt, black pepper, garlic powder, oregano, and red pepper flakes until well combined and the spices are incorporated. With your hands, form the mixture into 8 small patties about ½ inch thick.
2. Place a large skillet over medium heat. Add the ghee.
3. Add the turkey patties, working in batches if necessary. Cook for about 3 minutes per side until done. Serve immediately or refrigerate in a sealed container for up to 3 days.

PER SERVING

Calories: 159; Total Fat: 10g; Saturated Fat: 4g; Cholesterol: 60mg; Carbohydrates: 3g; Fiber: 0g; Protein: 16g

Chia-Cherry Oats

Prep time: 5 minutes, plus 25 minutes chilling| Serves 2

- 1¼ cups nut milk of choice
- ¼ cup plain whole-milk yogurt
- 1 cup quick cook oats
- 2 tablespoons chia seeds
- 8 fresh cherries, pitted and halved
- 2 tablespoons nut butter of choice
- ¼ teaspoon vanilla extract

1. In a large bowl, stir together the milk, yogurt, oats, chia seeds, cherries, nut butter, and vanilla until well combined.
2. Divide the mixture between 2 lidded jars. Seal and refrigerate for about 25 minutes.

PER SERVING

Calories: 564; Total Fat: 32g; Saturated Fat: 3g; Cholesterol: 4mg; Carbohydrates: 27g; Fiber: 13g; Protein: 22g

Banana Oat Pancakes

Prep time: 5 minutes | Cook time: 10 minutes| Serves 2

- 1 cup rolled oats
- 1 ripe banana
- 2 eggs
- 1 egg white
- 2 teaspoons ground cinnamon
- 1 teaspoon vanilla extract
- ½ teaspoon salt
- 1 tablespoon coconut oil, divided

1. In a food processor (or blender), grind the oats into a coarse flour. Add the banana, eggs, egg white, cinnamon, vanilla, and salt. Blend until a smooth batter forms.
2. In a small skillet over medium heat, heat ½ tablespoon of coconut oil. Spoon the batter into the pan to create pancakes of the desired size; cook in batches if necessary to avoid crowding. Cook for about 2 minutes until small bubbles form on the top. Flip and cook the other side for 1 to 2 minutes. Repeat with the remaining coconut oil and batter. Serve hot.

PER SERVING

Calories: 360; Total Fat: 15g; Saturated Fat: 8g; Cholesterol: 186mg; Carbohydrates: 17g; Fiber: 7g; Protein: 15g

Orange-Glazed Raspberry Muffins

Prep time: 5 minutes | Cook time: 40 minutes | Serves 6

- 2 eggs, beaten
- 2 cups whole-wheat flour
- 1½ tsp baking powder
- A pinch of sea salt
- 5 tbsp almond butter, softened
- 1 cup pure date sugar
- ½ cup oat milk
- 2 tsp vanilla extract
- 1 lemon, zested
- 1 cup dried raspberries
- 2 tbsp orange juice

1. Preheat your oven to 400°F. Grease 6 muffin cups with cooking spray. In a medium bowl, mix the flour, baking powder, and salt.
2. In another bowl, cream the almond butter, half of the date sugar, and eggs. Mix in the oat milk, vanilla, and lemon zest. Combine both mixtures, fold in raspberries, and fill muffin cups two-thirds way up with the batter. Bake for 20-25 minutes.
3. In a medium bowl, whisk orange juice and remaining date sugar until smooth.
4. Remove the muffins when ready and transfer to them a wire rack to cool. Drizzle the glaze on top. Serve.

PER SERVING

Cal 370; Fat 10g; Carbs 62g; Protein 10.2g

Almond Yogurt with Berries & Walnuts

Prep time: 5 minutes | Cook time: 10 minutes | Serves 4

- 4 cups almond milk
- 2 cups Greek yogurt
- 2 tbsp pure maple syrup
- 2 cups mixed berries
- ¼ cup chopped walnuts

1. In a medium bowl, mix the yogurt and maple syrup until well-combined.
2. Divide the mixture into 4 breakfast bowls. Top with the berries and walnuts. Enjoy immediately.

PER SERVING

Cal 703; Fat 63g; Carbs 32.1g; Protein 13g

Sweet Orange Crepes

Prep time: 5 minutes | Cook time: 30 minutes | Serves 4

- 2 eggs
- 1 tsp vanilla extract
- 1 tsp pure date sugar
- ¼ tsp sea salt
- 2 cups almond flour
- 1½ cups oat milk
- ½ cup melted coconut oil
- 3 tbsp fresh orange juice
- 3 tbsp olive oil

1. In a medium bowl, whisk the eggs with vanilla, date sugar, and salt. Pour in a quarter cup of almond flour and whisk, then a quarter cup of oat milk, and mix until no lumps remain.
2. Repeat the mixing process with the remaining almond flour and almond milk in the same quantities until exhausted. Mix in the coconut oil and orange juice until the mixture is runny, like pancakes.
3. Brush a nonstick skillet with some olive oil and place over medium heat. Pour 1 tablespoon of the batter into the pan and swirl the skillet quickly and all around to coat the pan with the batter. Cook until the batter is dry and golden brown beneath, about 30 seconds.
4. Use a spatula to flip the crepe and cook the other side until golden brown too. Fold the crepe onto a plate and set aside. Repeat making more crepes with the remaining batter until exhausted. Serve and enjoy!

PER SERVING

Cal 677; Fat 58g; Carbs 23g; Protein 16.4g

Coconut Oat Bread

Prep time: 5 minutes | Cook time: 50 minutes | Serves 4

- 4 cups whole-wheat flour
- ¼ tsp sea salt
- ½ cup rolled oats
- 1 tsp baking soda
- 1¾ cups coconut milk, thick
- 2 tbsp pure maple syrup

1. Preheat your oven to 450°F. In a bowl, mix flour, salt, oats, and baking soda. Add in coconut milk and maple syrup and whisk until dough forms.
2. Dust your hands with some flour and knead the dough into a ball. Shape the dough into a circle and place on a baking sheet.
3. Cut a deep cross on the dough and bake in the oven for 15 minutes. Reduce the heat to 400°F and bake further for 20-25 minutes or until a hollow sound is made when the bottom of the bread is tapped. Slice and serve.

PER SERVING

Cal 761; Fat 27g; Carbs 115g; Protein 17g

Spicy Quinoa Bowl with Black Beans

Prep time: 5 minutes | Cook time: 25 minutes | Serves 4

- 1 cup brown quinoa, rinsed
- 3 tbsp Greek yogurt
- ½ lime, juiced
- 2 tbsp chopped cilantro
- 1 cup canned black beans
- 3 tbsp tomato salsa
- ¼ avocado, sliced
- 2 radishes, shredded
- 1 tbsp pepitas

1. Cook the quinoa with 2 cups of salted water in a pot over medium heat or until the liquid absorbs, 15 minutes.
2. Spoon the quinoa into serving bowls and fluff with a fork. In a small bowl, mix the yogurt, lime juice, cilantro, and salt.
3. Divide this mixture on the quinoa and top with beans, salsa, avocado, radishes, and pepitas. Serve.

PER SERVING

Cal 340; Fat 9g; Carbs 49g; Protein 19.1g

Pecan & Pumpkin Seed Oat Jars

Prep time: 5 minutes | Cook time: 10 minutes + chilling time | Serves 4

- 2½ cups old-fashioned rolled oats
- 5 tbsp pumpkin seeds
- 5 tbsp chopped pecans
- 5 cups soy milk
- 2½ tsp maple syrup
- Sea salt to taste
- 1 tsp ground cardamom
- 1 tsp ground ginger

1. In a bowl, put oats, pumpkin seeds, pecans, soy milk, maple syrup, salt, cardamom, and ginger; toss to combine.
2. Divide the mixture between mason jars. Seal the lids and place the jars in the fridge for about 10 hours. Serve.

PER SERVING

Cal 441; Fat 16g; Carbs 59g; Protein 18.4g

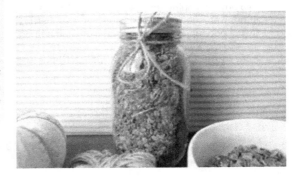

Simple Apple Muffins

Prep time: 5 minutes | Cook time: 40 minutes | Serves 6

- 1 egg
- 2 cups whole-wheat flour
- 1 cup pure date sugar
- 2 tsp baking powder
- ¼ tsp sea salt
- 2 tsp cinnamon powder
- 1/3 cup melted coconut oil
- 1/3 cup almond milk
- 2 apples, chopped
- ½ cup almond butter, cubed

1. Preheat your oven to 400°F. Grease 6 muffin cups with cooking spray. In a bowl, mix 1½ cups of whole-wheat flour, ¾ cup of the date sugar, baking powder, salt, and 1 tsp of cinnamon powder.
2. Whisk in the melted coconut oil, egg, and almond milk and fold in the apples. Fill the muffin cups two-thirds way up with the batter.
3. In a bowl, mix the remaining flour, remaining date sugar, and cold almond butter. Top the muffin batter with the mixture. Bake for 20 minutes.
4. Remove the muffins onto a wire rack, allow cooling, and dust them with the remaining cinnamon powder. Serve and enjoy!

PER SERVING

Cal 463; Fat 18g; Carbs 71g; Protein 8.2g

Blueberry Muesli Breakfast

Prep time: 5 minutes | Cook time: 10 minutes | Serves 4

- 2 cups spelt flakes
- 2 cups puffed cereal
- ¼ cup sunflower seeds
- ¼ cup almonds
- ¼ cup raisins
- ¼ cup dried cranberries
- ¼ cup chopped dried figs
- ¼ cup shredded coconut
- ¼ cup dark chocolate chips
- 3 tsp ground cinnamon
- ½ cup coconut milk
- ½ cup blueberries

1. In a bowl, combine the spelt flakes, puffed cereal, sunflower seeds, almonds, raisins, cranberries, figs, coconut, chocolate chips, and cinnamon. Toss to mix well.
2. Pour in the coconut milk. Let sit for 1 hour and serve topped with blueberries.

PER SERVING

Cal 333; Fat 15g; Carbs 49g; Protein 6.2g

Chocolate-Mango Quinoa Bowl

Prep time: 5 minutes | Cook time: 35 minutes | Serves 2

- 1 cup quinoa
- 1 tsp ground cinnamon
- 1 cup non-dairy milk
- 1 large mango, chopped
- 3 tbsp cocoa powder
- 2 tbsp almond butter
- 1 tbsp hemp seeds
- 1 tbsp walnuts
- ¼ cup raspberries

1. In a pot, combine the quinoa, cinnamon, milk, and 1 cup of water over medium heat. Bring to a boil, low heat, and simmer covered for 25-30 minutes.
2. In a bowl, mash the mango and mix cocoa powder, almond butter, and hemp seeds. In a serving bowl, place cooked quinoa and mango mixture. Top with walnuts and raspberries. Serve.

PER SERVING

Cal 584; Fat 21g; Carbs 83g; Protein 23.4g

Orange-Carrot Muffins with Cherries

Prep time: 5 minutes | Cook time: 45 minutes | Serves 6

- 1 tsp avocado oil
- 2 tbsp almond butter
- ¼ cup non-dairy milk
- 1 orange, peeled
- 1 carrot, coarsely chopped
- 3 tbsp molasses
- 2 tbsp ground flaxseed
- 1 tsp apple cider vinegar
- 1 tsp pure vanilla extract
- ½ tsp ground cinnamon
- ½ tsp ground ginger
- ¼ tsp ground nutmeg
- ¼ tsp allspice
- ¾ cup whole-wheat flour
- 1 tsp baking powder
- ½ tsp baking soda
- ½ cup rolled oats
- 2 tbsp raisins
- 2 tbsp sunflower seeds

1. Preheat your oven to 350°F. Grease 6 muffin cups with avocado oil. In a food processor, add the almond butter, milk, orange, carrot, cherries, molasses, flaxseed, vinegar, vanilla, cinnamon, ginger, nutmeg, and allspice and blend until smooth.
2. In a bowl, combine the flour, baking powder, and baking soda. Fold in the wet mixture and gently stir to combine. Mix in the oats, raisins, and sunflower seeds. Divide the batter between muffin cups. Put in a baking tray and bake for 30 minutes.

PER SERVING

Cal 210; Fat 5g; Carbs 36.6g; Protein 5.3g

Lemony Quinoa Muffins
Prep time: 5 minutes | Cook time: 25 minutes | Serves 4

- 2 tbsp coconut oil melted
- ¼ cup ground flaxseed
- 2 cups lemon curd
- ½ cup pure date sugar
- 1 tsp apple cider vinegar
- 2 ½ cups whole-wheat flour
- 1 ½ cups cooked quinoa
- 2 tsp baking soda
- A pinch of sea salt
- ½ cup raisins

1. Preheat your oven to 400°F. In a bowl, combine the flaxseed and ½ cup water. Stir in the lemon curd, sugar, coconut oil, and vinegar.
2. Add in flour, quinoa, baking soda, and salt. Put in the raisins, be careful not too fluffy.
3. Divide the batter between greased muffin tin and bake for 20 minutes until golden and set. Allow cooling slightly before removing it from the tin. Serve.

PER SERVING

Cal 719; Fat 11g; Carbs 133g; Protein 19g

Morning Pecan & Pear Farro
Prep time: 5 minutes | Cook time: 20 minutes | Serves 4

- 1 cup farro
- 1 tbsp peanut butter
- 2 pears, peeled and chopped
- ¼ cup chopped pecans

1. Bring salted water to a boil in a pot over high heat. Stir in farro. Lower the heat, cover, and simmer for 15 minutes until the farro is tender and the liquid has absorbed.
2. Turn the heat off and add in the peanut butter, pears, and pecans. Cover and rest for 12-15 minutes. Serve.

PER SERVING

Cal 387; Fat 28g; Carbs 32g; Protein 8.6g

Almond Oatmeal Porridge
Prep time: 5 minutes | Cook time: 25 minutes | Serves 4

- 2 cups old-fashioned rolled oats
- 2 ½ cups vegetable broth
- 2 ½ cups almond milk
- ½ cup steel-cut oats
- 1 tbsp pearl barley
- ½ cup slivered almonds
- ¼ cup nutritional yeast

1. Pour the broth and almond milk in a pot over medium heat and bring to a boil. Stir in oats, pearl barley, almond slivers, and nutritional yeast.
2. Reduce the heat and simmer for 20 minutes. Add in the oats, cook for an additional 5 minutes, until creamy. Allow cooling before serving.

PER SERVING

Cal 619; Fat 45g; Carbs 44g; Protein 15.4g

Classic Walnut Waffles with Maple Syrup
Prep time: 5 minutes | Cook time: 15 minutes | Serves 4

- 1 ¾ cups whole-wheat flour
- ⅓ cup ground walnuts
- 1 tbsp baking powder
- 1 ½ cups soy milk
- 3 tbsp pure maple syrup
- 3 tbsp coconut oil, melted

1. Preheat your waffle iron and grease with oil. Combine flour, walnuts, baking powder, and salt in a bowl. In another bowl, mix the milk and coconut oil.
2. Pour into the walnut mixture and whisk until well combined. Spoon a ladleful of the batter onto the waffle iron. Cook for 3-5 minutes, until golden brown. Repeat the process until no batter is left. Top with maple syrup to serve.

PER SERVING

Cal 440; Fat 18g; Carbs 58g; Protein 11.4g

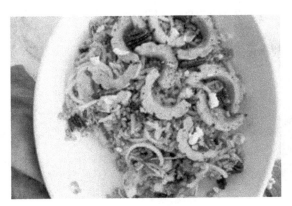

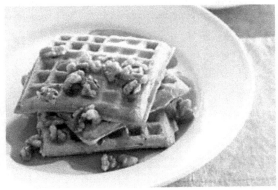

Tangerine Banana Toast

Prep time: 5 minutes | Cook time: 25 minutes | Serves 4

- 3 bananas
- 1 cup almond milk
- Zest and juice of 1 tangerine
- 1 tsp ground cinnamon
- ¼ tsp grated nutmeg
- 4 whole-wheat bread slices
- 1 tbsp olive oil

1. Blend the bananas, almond milk, tangerine juice, tangerine zest, cinnamon, and nutmeg until smooth in a food processor. Spread into a baking dish.
2. Submerge the bread slices in the mixture for 3-4 minutes. Heat the oil in a skillet over medium heat. Fry the bread for 5 minutes until golden brown. Serve hot.

PER SERVING

Cal 316; Fat 19g; Carbs 35g; Protein 6g

Coconut Blueberry Muffins

Prep time: 5 minutes | Cook time: 30 minutes | Serves 6

- 1 tbsp coconut oil, melted
- 1 cup quick-cooking oats
- 1 cup boiling water
- ½ cup almond milk
- ¼ cup ground flaxseed
- 1 tsp almond extract
- 1 tsp apple cider vinegar
- 1½ cups whole-wheat flour
- ½ cup pure date sugar
- 2 tsp baking soda
- A pinch of sea salt
- 1 cup blueberries

1. Preheat your oven to 400°F. In a bowl, stir oats with boiling water until they are softened.
2. Pour in the coconut oil, milk, flaxseed, almond extract, and vinegar. Add the flour, date sugar, baking soda, and salt. Gently stir in blueberries. Divide the batter between greased muffins.
3. Bake for 20 minutes until lightly brown. Allow cooling for 10 minutes. Using a spatula, run the sides of the muffins to take out. Serve and enjoy!

PER SERVING

Cal 317; Fat 10g; Carbs 50.6g; Protein 7g

Orange-Bran Cups with Dates

Prep time: 5 minutes | Cook time: 30 minutes | Serves 6

- 1 tsp avocado oil
- 3 cups bran flakes cereal
- 1½ cups whole-wheat flour
- ½ cup dates, chopped
- 3 tsp baking powder
- ½ tsp ground cinnamon
- ½ tsp sea salt
- ⅓ cup brown sugar
- ¾ cup fresh orange juice

1. Preheat your oven to 400°F. Grease a 12-cup muffin tin with avocado oil. Mix the bran flakes, flour, dates, baking powder, cinnamon, and salt in a bowl.
2. In another bowl, combine the sugar and orange juice until blended. Pour into the dry mixture and whisk.
3. Divide the mixture between the cups of the muffin tin. Bake for 20 minutes or until golden brown and set. Cool for a few minutes before removing from the tin and serve.

PER SERVING

Cal 256; Fat 1g; Carbs 57g; Protein 5.8g

Scrambled Tofu with Swiss Chard

Prep time: 5 minutes | Cook time: 35 minutes | Serves 4

- 1 (14-oz) package tofu, crumbled
- 2 tsp olive oil
- 1 onion, chopped
- 3 cloves minced garlic
- 1 celery stalk, chopped
- 2 large carrots, chopped
- 1 tsp chili powder
- ½ tsp ground cumin
- ½ tsp ground turmeric
- Sea salt and pepper to taste
- 5 cups Swiss chard

1. Heat the oil in a skillet over medium heat. Add in the onion, garlic, celery, and carrots. Sauté for 5 minutes.
2. Stir in tofu, chili powder, cumin, turmeric, salt, and pepper, cook for 7-8 minutes more. Mix in Swiss chard and cook until wilted, 3 minutes. Allow cooling and seal, and serve.

PER SERVING

Cal 128; Fat 7g; Carbs 10.5g; Protein 9.7g

Spicy Apple Pancakes

Prep time: 5 minutes | Cook time: 30 minutes | Serves 4

- 2 cups almond milk
- 1 tsp apple cider vinegar
- 2 ½ cups whole-wheat flour
- 2 tbsp baking powder
- ½ tsp baking soda
- 1 tsp sea salt
- ½ tsp ground cinnamon
- ¼ tsp grated nutmeg
- ¼ tsp ground allspice
- ½ cup sugar-free applesauce
- 1 tbsp coconut oil

1. Whisk the almond milk and apple cider vinegar in a bowl and set aside. In another bowl, combine the flour, baking powder, baking soda, salt, cinnamon, nutmeg, and allspice.
2. Transfer the almond mixture to another bowl and beat with the applesauce and 1 cup of water. Pour in the dry ingredients and stir. Melt some coconut oil in a skillet over medium heat.
3. Pour a ladle of the batter and cook for 5 minutes, flipping once until golden. Repeat the process until the batter is exhausted. Serve.

PER SERVING

Cal 596; Fat 33g; Carbs 67.2g; Protein 11g

Yogurt, Berry, and Walnut Parfait

Prep time: 5 minutes | Cook time: 5 minutes | Serves 2

- 2 cups plain unsweetened yogurt, or plain unsweetened coconut yogurt or almond yogurt
- 2 tablespoons honey
- 1 cup fresh blueberries
- 1 cup fresh raspberries
- ½ cup walnut pieces

1. In a medium bowl, whisk the yogurt and honey. Spoon into 2 serving bowls.
2. Top each with ½ cup blueberries, ½ cup raspberries, and ¼ cup walnut pieces.

PER SERVING

Calories: 505; Total Fat: 22g; Total Carbs: 56g; Sugar: 45g; Fiber: 8g; Protein: 23g; Sodium: 174mg

Oatmeal and Cinnamon with Dried Cranberries

Prep time: 5 minutes | Cook time: 8 minutes | Serves 2

- 1 cup water
- 1 cup almond milk
- pinch sea salt
- 1 cup old-fashioned oats
- ½ cup dried cranberries
- 1 teaspoon ground cinnamon

1. In a medium saucepan over high heat, bring the water, almond milk, and salt to a boil.
2. Stir in the oats, cranberries, and cinnamon. Reduce the heat to medium and cook for 5 minutes, stirring occasionally.
3. Remove the oatmeal from the heat. Cover the pot and let it stand for 3 minutes. Stir before serving.

PER SERVING

Calories: 101; Total Fat: 2g; Total Carbs: 18g; Sugar: 1g; Fiber: 4g; Protein: 3g; Sodium: 126mg

Spinach Frittata

Prep time: 5 minutes | Cook time: 15 minutes | Serves 4

- 2 tablespoons extra-virgin olive oil
- 2 cups fresh baby spinach
- 8 eggs, beaten
- 1 teaspoon garlic powder
- ½ teaspoon sea salt
- ¼ teaspoon freshly ground black pepper
- 2 tablespoons grated parmesan cheese

1. Preheat the broiler to high.
2. In a large ovenproof skillet (well-seasoned cast iron works well) over medium-high heat, heat the olive oil until it shimmers.
3. Add the spinach and cook for about 3 minutes, stirring occasionally.
4. In a medium bowl, whisk the eggs, garlic powder, salt, and pepper. Carefully pour the egg mixture over the spinach and cook the eggs for about 3 minutes until they begin to set around the edges.
5. Using a rubber spatula, gently pull the eggs away from the edges of the pan. Tilt the pan to let the uncooked egg flow into the edges. Cook for 2 to 3 minutes until the edges set.
6. Sprinkle with the Parmesan cheese and put the skillet under the broiler. Broil for about 3 minutes until the top puffs.
7. Cut into wedges to serve.

PER SERVING

Calories: 203; Total Fat: 17g; Total Carbs: 2g; Sugar: <1g; Fiber: <1g; Protein: 13g; Sodium: 402mg

Mushroom and Bell Pepper Omelet

Prep time: 5 minutes | Cook time: 15 minutes| Serves 2

- 2 tablespoons extra-virgin olive oil
- 1 red bell pepper, sliced
- 1 cup mushrooms, sliced
- 6 eggs, beaten
- ½ teaspoon sea salt
- ⅛ teaspoon freshly ground black pepper

1. In a large nonstick skillet over medium-high heat, heat the olive oil until it shimmers.
2. Add the red bell pepper and mushrooms. Cook for about 4 minutes, stirring occasionally, until soft.
3. In a medium bowl, whisk the eggs, salt, and pepper. Pour the eggs over the vegetables and cook for about 3 minutes without stirring until the eggs begin to set around the edges.
4. Using a rubber spatula, gently pull the eggs away from the edges of the pan. Tilt the pan so the uncooked egg can flow to the edges. Cook for 2 to 3 minutes until the eggs are set at the edges and the center.
5. Using a spatula, fold the omelet in half. Cut into wedges to serve.

PER SERVING

Calories: 336; Total Fat: 27g; Total Carbs: 7g; Sugar: 5g; Fiber: 1g; Protein: 18g; Sodium: 656mg

Smoked Salmon Scrambled Eggs

Prep time: 5 minutes | Cook time: 8 minutes| Serves 4

- 2 tablespoons extra-virgin olive oil
- 6 ounces smoked salmon, flaked
- 8 eggs, beaten
- ¼ teaspoon freshly ground black pepper

1. In a large nonstick skillet over medium-high heat, heat the olive oil until it shimmers.
2. Add the salmon and cook for 3 minutes, stirring.
3. In a medium bowl, whisk the eggs and pepper. Add them to the skillet and cook for about 5 minutes, stirring gently, until done.

PER SERVING

Calories: 236; Total Fat: 18g; Total Carbs: <1g; Sugar: <1g; Fiber: 0g; Protein: 19g; Sodium: 974mg

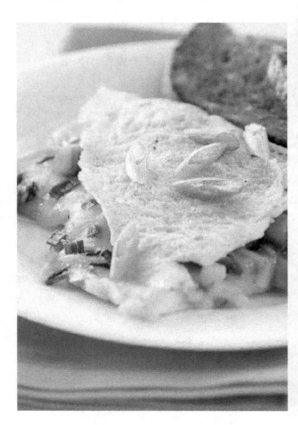

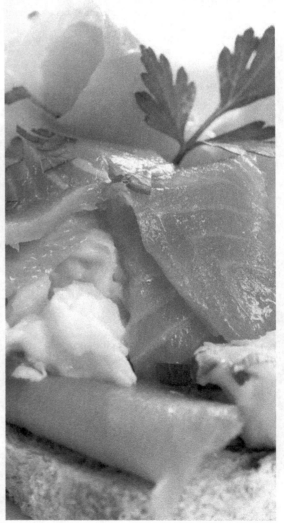

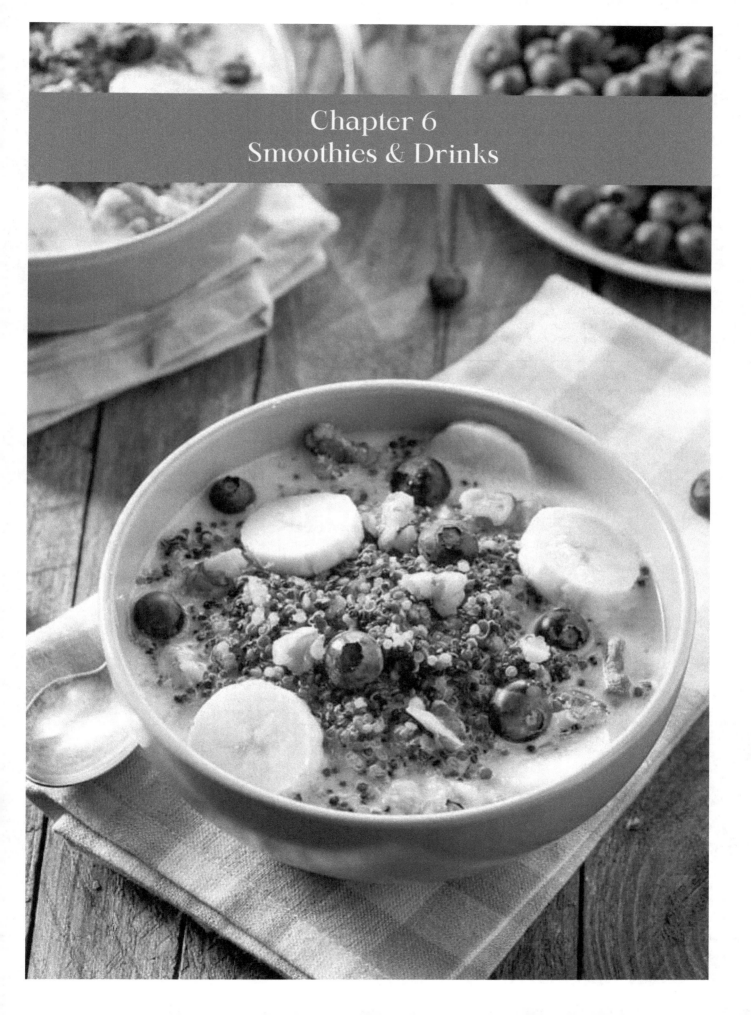

Chapter 6
Smoothies & Drinks

Inflammation-Soothing Smoothie
Prep time: 5 minutes | Cook time: 5 minutes| Serves 1

- 1 pear, cored and quartered
- ½ fennel bulb
- 1 thin slice fresh ginger
- 1 cup packed spinach
- ½ cucumber, peeled if wax-coated or not organic
- ½ cup water
- Ice (optional)

1. In a blender, combine the pear, fennel, ginger, spinach, cucumber, water, and ice (if using). Blend until smooth.

PER SERVING

Calories: 147; Total Fat: 1g;Total Carbohydrates: 37g;Sugar: 6g; Fiber: 9g;Protein: 4g; Sodium: 89mg

Eat-Your-Vegetables Smoothie
Prep time: 5 minutes | Cook time: 5 minutes| Serves 1

- 1 carrot, trimmed
- 1 small beet, scrubbed and quartered
- 1 celery stalk
- ½ cup fresh raspberries
- 1 cup coconut water
- 1 teaspoon balsamic vinegar
- Ice (optional)

1. In a blender, combine the carrot, beet, celery, raspberries, coconut water, balsamic vinegar, and ice (if using). Blend until smooth.

PER SERVING

Calories: 140; Total Fat: 1g;Total Carbohydrates: 24g;Sugar: 23g; Fiber: 8g;Protein: 3g; Sodium: 293mg

Cherry Smoothie
Prep time: 5 minutes | Cook time: 5 minutes| Serves 1

- 1 cup frozen no-added-sugar pitted cherries
- ¼ cup fresh, or frozen, raspberries
- ¾ cup coconut water
- 1 tablespoon raw honey or maple syrup
- 1 teaspoon chia seeds
- 1 teaspoon hemp seeds
- Drop vanilla extract
- Ice (optional)

1. In a blender, combine the cherries, raspberries, coconut water, honey, chia seeds, hemp seeds, vanilla, and ice (if using). Blend until smooth.

PER SERVING

Calories: 266; Total Fat: 2g;Total Carbohydrates: 52g;Sugar: 48g; Fiber: 6g;Protein: 3g; Sodium: 122mg

Green Apple Smoothie
Prep time: 5 minutes | Cook time: 5 minutes| Serves 1

- ½ cup coconut water
- 1 green apple, cored, seeded, and quartered
- 1 cup spinach
- ¼ lemon, seeded
- ½ cucumber, peeled and seeded
- 2 teaspoons raw honey, or maple syrup
- Ice (optional)

1. In a blender, combine the coconut water, apple, spinach, lemon, cucumber, honey, and ice (if using). Blend until smooth.

PER SERVING

Calories: 176; Total Fat: 1g;Total Carbohydrates: 41g;Sugar: 34g; Fiber: 6g;Protein: 2g; Sodium: 110mg

One-for-All Smoothie
Prep time: 5 minutes | Cook time: 5 minutes| Serves 1

- 1 cup packed spinach
- ½ cup fresh blueberries
- ½ banana
- 1 cup coconut milk
- ½ teaspoon vanilla extract

1. In a blender, combine the spinach, blueberries, banana, coconut milk, and vanilla. Blend until smooth.

PER SERVING

Calories: 152; Total Fat: 5g;Total Carbohydrates: 27g;Sugar: 15g; Fiber: 5g;Protein: 2g; Sodium: 90mg

Mango-Thyme Smoothie
Prep time: 5 minutes | Cook time: 5 minutes| Serves 1

- 1 cup fresh or frozen mango chunks
- ½ cup fresh seedless green grapes
- ¼ fennel bulb
- ½ cup unsweetened almond milk
- ½ teaspoon fresh thyme leaves
- Pinch sea salt
- Pinch freshly ground black pepper
- Ice (optional)

1. In a blender, combine the mango, grapes, fennel, almond milk, thyme leaves, sea salt, pepper, and ice (if using). Blend until smooth.

PER SERVING

Calories: 274; Total Fat: 4g;Total Carbohydrates: 65g;Sugar: 54g; Fiber: 7g;Protein: 3g; Sodium: 125mg

Year-Round Pumpkin Pie Smoothie

Prep time: 5 minutes| Serves 2

- 1 banana
- ½ cup unsweetened canned pumpkin
- 1 cup nut milk of choice
- 2 or 3 ice cubes
- 2 heaping tablespoons almond butter
- 1 teaspoon ground cinnamon
- 1 teaspoon ground nutmeg
- 1 teaspoon pure maple syrup
- 1 teaspoon vanilla extract

1. In a blender, combine the banana, pumpkin, nut milk, ice, almond butter, cinnamon, nutmeg, maple syrup, and vanilla until smooth.
2. Pour into two tall glasses and serve immediately.

PER SERVING

Calories: 235; Total Fat: 11g; Saturated Fat: 0.6g; Cholesterol: 0mg; Carbohydrates: 27.8g; Fiber: 6.9g; Protein: 5.6g

Protein Powerhouse Smoothie

Prep time: 5 minutes | Cook time: 5 minutes| Serves 1

- 1 cup packed kale leaves, thoroughly washed
- ¼ avocado
- 1 cup fresh grapes
- ¼ cup cashews (optional)
- 1 tablespoon hemp seed
- 1 cup coconut milk
- Ice (optional)

1. In a blender, combine the kale, avocado, grapes, cashews (if using), hemp seed, mint leaves, coconut milk, and ice (if using). Blend until smooth.

PER SERVING

Calories: 500; Total Fat: 32g;Total Carbohydrates: 47g;Sugar: 34g; Fiber: 7g;Protein: 13g; Sodium: 199mg

Chai Smoothie

Prep time: 5 minutes | Cook time: 5 minutes| Serves 1

- 1 cup unsweetened almond milk
- 1 date, pitted and chopped
- ¼ teaspoon vanilla extract
- ½ teaspoon chai spice blend
- Pinch salt
- 1 banana, sliced into ¼-inch rounds
- Ice cubes

1. In a blender, combine the almond milk, date, vanilla, chai spice blend, salt, banana, and ice. Blend until smooth.

PER SERVING

Calories: 171; Total Fat: 4g;Total Carbohydrates: 35g;Sugar: 20g; Fiber: 5g;Protein: 3g; Sodium: 336mg

Peachy Mint Punch

Prep time: 5 minutes | Cook time: 15 minutes| Serves 2

- 1 (10-ounce) bag frozen no-added-sugar peach slices, thawed
- 3 tablespoons freshly squeezed lemon juice
- 3 tablespoons raw honey or maple syrup
- 1 tablespoon lemon zest
- 2 cups coconut water
- 2 cups sparkling water
- 4 fresh mint sprigs, divided
- Ice

1. In a food processor, combine the peaches, lemon juice, honey, and lemon zest. Process until smooth.
2. In a large pitcher, stir together the peach purée and coconut water. Chill the mixture in the refrigerator.
3. When ready to serve, fill four large (16-ounce) glasses with ice. Add 1 mint sprig to each glass. Add about ¾ cup peach mixture to each glass and top each with sparkling water.

PER SERVING

Calories: 81; Total Fat: 0g;Total Carbohydrates: 18g;Sugar: 14g; Fiber: 1g;Protein: 0g; Sodium: 85mg

Pineapple-Carrot-Ginger Juice

Prep time: 10 minutes| Serves 2

- 3 cups chopped fresh pineapple
- 8 carrots, roughly chopped
- ¼ cup filtered water
- 1 (1-inch) piece peeled fresh ginger
- Ice, for serving

1. In a blender, blend the pineapple, carrots, water, and ginger until smooth.
2. Place a nut milk bag or piece of cheesecloth over the top of a medium bowl. Pour the juice into the mesh material. Squeeze the juice through the material until all the liquid has drained into the bowl. Discard the solids. In two tall glasses, add ice and serve immediately.

PER SERVING

Calories: 135; Total Fat: 0.7g; Saturated Fat: 0.1g; Cholesterol: 0mg; Carbohydrates: 40g; Fiber: 1g; Protein: 2.6g

Green Tea and Pear Smoothie

Prep time: 5 minutes | Cook time: 5 minutes| Serves 1

- 2 cups strongly brewed green tea
- 2 pears, peeled, cored, and chopped
- 2 tablespoons honey
- 1 (1-inch) piece fresh ginger, peeled and roughly chopped, or 1 teaspoon ground ginger
- 1 cup unsweetened almond milk
- 1 cup crushed ice

1. In a blender, combine the green tea, pears, honey, ginger, almond milk, and ice. Blend until smooth.

PER SERVING

Calories: 208; Total Fat: 2g; Total Carbs: 51g; Sugar: 38g; Fiber: 7g; Protein: 1g; Sodium: 94mg

Tart Cherry Sparkling Lemonade

Prep time: 5 minutes| Serves 1

- 8 ounces sparkling mineral water
- 4 ounces tart cherry juice
- 2 tablespoons freshly squeezed lemon juice
- Few drops raw honey (optional)
- Ice, for serving

1. In a tall glass, gently stir together the mineral water, cherry juice, lemon juice, and honey (if using). Add ice and serve.

PER SERVING

Calories: 137; Total Fat: 0.1g; Saturated Fat: 0g; Cholesterol: 0mg; Carbohydrates: 34.1g; Fiber: 0.1g; Protein: 1.1g

Matcha Berry Smoothie

Prep time: 5 minutes| Serves 2

- 2 cups nut milk of choice
- 2 cups frozen blueberries
- 1 banana
- 2 tablespoons neutral-flavored protein powder (optional)
- 1 tablespoon matcha powder
- 1 tablespoon chia seeds
- ¼ teaspoon ground cinnamon
- ¼ teaspoon ground ginger
- Pinch salt

1. In a blender, blend the nut milk, blueberries, banana, protein powder (if using), matcha, chia seeds, cinnamon, ginger, and salt until smooth. Pour into two glasses and serve immediately.

PER SERVING(WITHOUT PROTEIN POWDER)

Calories: 208; Total Fat: 5.7g; Saturated Fat: 0.3g; Cholesterol: 0mg; Carbohydrates: 31g; Fiber: 8.3g; Protein: 8.7g

Turmeric and Green Tea Mango Smoothie

Prep time: 5 minutes | Cook time: 5 minutes| Serves 2

2 cups cubed mango
2 teaspoons turmeric powder
2 tablespoons matcha powder(green tea)
2 tablespoons honey
1 cup crushed ice

1. In a blender, combine the mango, turmeric, matcha, almond milk, honey, and ice. Blend until smooth.

PER SERVING

Calories: 285; Total Fat: 3g; Total Carbs: 68g; Sugar: 63g; Fiber: 6g; Protein: 4g; Sodium: 94mg

Sweet Fig Smoothie

Prep time: 5 minutes| Serves 2

- 7 whole figs, fresh or frozen, halved
- 1 banana
- 1 cup plain whole-milk yogurt
- 1 cup almond milk
- 1 tablespoon almond butter
- 1 teaspoon ground flaxseed
- 1 teaspoon raw honey
- Ice (optional)

1. In a blender, combine the figs, banana, yogurt, almond milk, almond butter, flaxseed, and honey. Blend until smooth.
2. Add ice (if using) and blend again to thicken. Pour into two tall glasses and serve immediately.

PER SERVING

Calories: 362; Total Fat: 12g; Saturated Fat: 3g; Cholesterol: 16mg; Carbohydrates: 60g; Fiber: 9g; Protein: 9g

Coconut-Ginger Smoothie

Prep time: 5 minutes | Cook time: 5 minutes| Serves 1

- ½ cup coconut milk
- ½ cup coconut water
- ¼ avocado
- ¼ cup unsweetened coconut shreds or flakes
- 1 teaspoon raw honey or maple syrup
- 1 thin slice fresh ginger
- Pinch ground cardamom (optional)
- Ice (optional)

1. In a blender, combine the coconut milk, coconut water, avocado, coconut, honey, ginger, cardamom (if using), and ice (if using). Blend until smooth.

PER SERVING

Calories: 238; Total Fat: 18g;Total Carbohydrates: 16g;Sugar: 14g; Fiber: 10g;Protein: 5g; Sodium: 373mg

Kale and Banana Smoothie

Prep time: 5 minutes | Cook time: 5 minutes| Serves 1

- 2 cups unsweetened almond milk
- 2 cups kale, stemmed, leaves chopped
- 2 bananas, peeled
- 1 to 2 packets stevia, or to taste
- 1 teaspoon ground cinnamon
- 1 cup crushed ice

1. In a blender, combine the almond milk, kale, bananas, stevia, cinnamon, and ice.
2. Blend until smooth.

PER SERVING

Calories: 181; Total Fat: 4g; Total Carbs: 37g; Sugar: 15g; Fiber: 6g; Protein: 4g; Sodium: 210mg

Carrot-Strawberry Smoothie

Prep time: 5 minutes | Cook time: 5 minutes | Serves 2

- 1 cup diced carrots
- 1 cup strawberries
- 1 apple, chopped
- 2 tbsp maple syrup
- 2 cups almond milk

1. Place in a food processor all the ingredients. Blitz until smooth. Pour in glasses and serve.

PER SERVING

Cal 708; Fat 58g; Carbs 53.4g; Protein 7g

Ginger-Berry Smoothie

Prep time: 5 minutes | Cook time: 5 minutes| Serves 1

- 2 cups fresh blackberries
- 2 cups unsweetened almond milk
- 1 to 2 packets stevia, or to taste
- 1 (1-inch) piece fresh ginger, peeled and roughly chopped
- 2 cups crushed ice

1. In a blender, combine the blackberries, almond milk, stevia, ginger, and ice. Blend until smooth.

PER SERVING

Calories: 95; Total Fat: 3g; Total Carbs: 16g; Sugar: 7g; Fiber: 9g; Protein: 3g; Sodium: 152mg

Green Tea and Ginger Shake

Prep time: 5 minutes | Cook time: 5 minutes| Serves 2

- 2 tablespoons grated ginger
- 2 tablespoons honey
- 2 tablespoons matcha powder(green tea)
- 2 scoops low-fat vanilla ice cream
- 2 cups skim milk

1. In a blender, combine the ginger, honey, matcha, ice cream, and milk.
2. Blend until smooth.

PER SERVING

Calories: 340; Total Fat: 7g; Total Carbs: 56g; Sugar: 50g; Fiber: 2g; Protein: 11g; Sodium: 186mg

Tropical Smoothie Bowl

Prep time: 5 minutes | Cook time: 10 minutes | Serves 4

- 4 bananas, sliced
- 1 cup papaya, chopped
- 1 cup granola, crushed
- 2 cups fresh raspberries
- ½ cup slivered almonds
- 4 cups coconut milk

1. Put bananas, raspberries, and coconut milk in a food processor and pulse until smooth.
2. Transfer to a bowl and stir in granola. Top with almonds. Serve and enjoy!

PER SERVING

Cal 840; Fat 78g; Carbs 86g; Protein 19.3g

Blueberry, Chocolate, and Turmeric Smoothie

Prep time: 5 minutes | Cook time: 5 minutes| Serves 1

- 2 cups unsweetened almond milk
- 1 cup frozen wild blueberries
- 2 tablespoons cocoa powder
- 1 to 2 packets stevia, or to taste
- 1 (1-inch) piece fresh turmeric, peeled
- 1 cup crushed ice

1. In a blender, combine the almond milk, blueberries, cocoa powder, stevia, turmeric, and ice. Blend until smooth.

PER SERVING

Calories: 97; Total Fat: 5g; Total Carbs: 16g; Sugar: 7g; Fiber: 5g; Protein: 3g; Sodium: 182mg

Green Smoothie

Prep time: 5 minutes | Cook time: 5 minutes| Serves 1

- 3 cups baby spinach
- ¼ cup cilantro leaves
- 2 pears, peeled, cored, and chopped
- 3 cups unsweetened apple juice
- 1 tablespoon grated ginger
- 1 cup crushed ice

1. In a blender, combine the spinach, cilantro, pears, apple juice, ginger, and ice. Blend until smooth.

PER SERVING

Calories: 308; Total Fat: <1g; Total Carbs: 77g; Sugar: 61g; Fiber: 8g; Protein: 2g; Sodium: 50mg

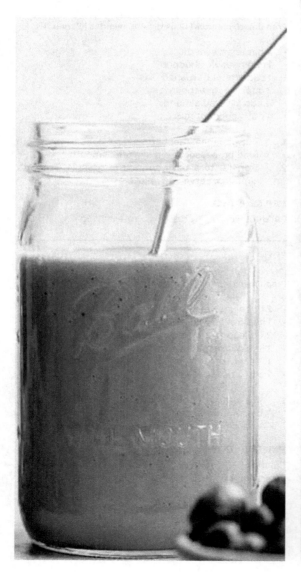

Super Green Smoothie

Prep time: 5 minutes | Cook time: 5 minutes| Serves 1

- 1 cup packed spinach
- ½ cucumber, peeled
- ½ pear
- ¼ avocado
- 1 teaspoon raw honey or maple syrup
- 1 cup unsweetened almond milk
- 2 mint leaves
- Pinch salt
- ½ lemon
- Ice (optional)

1. In a blender, combine the spinach, cucumber, pear, avocado, honey, almond milk, mint leaves, salt, 1 or 2 squeezes of lemon juice, and the ice (if using). Blend until smooth.

PER SERVING

Calories: 248; Total Fat: 14g;Total Carbohydrates: 33g;Sugar: 14g; Fiber: 10g;Protein: 5g; Sodium: 373mg

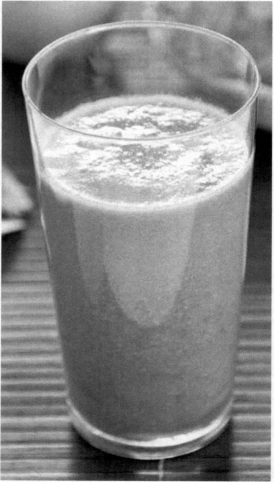

Chapter 7
Poultry

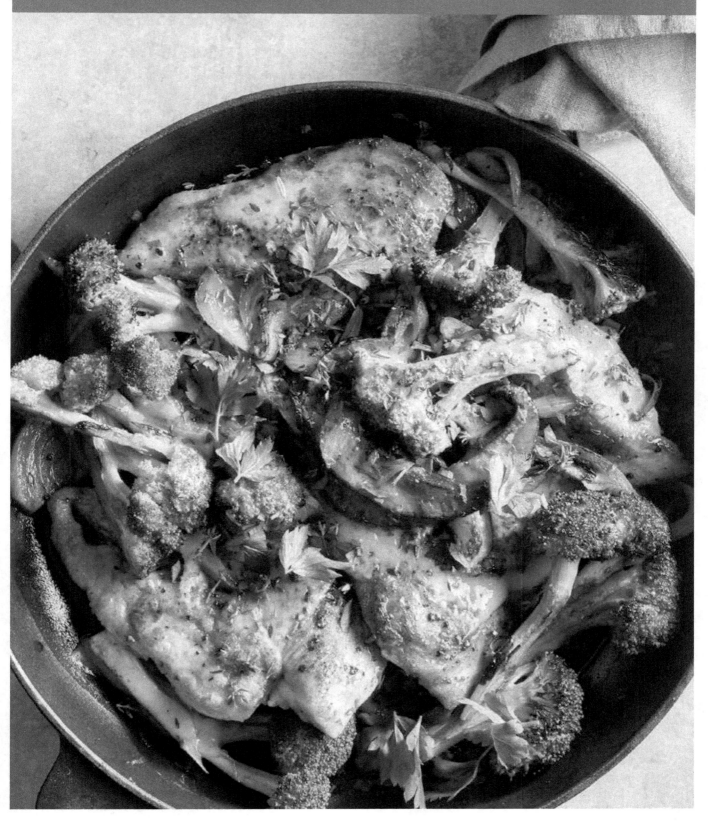

Sumac Chicken Thighs

Prep time: 5 minutes | Cook time: 55 minutes | Serves 4

- 6 bone-in chicken thighs
- 2 sweet potatoes, cubed
- 2 tbsp extra-virgin olive oil
- 2 shallots, sliced thin
- Sea salt and pepper to taste
- 1 tsp sumac
- ½ tsp ground cinnamon
- 1 cup chicken broth

1. Preheat your oven to 425°F. In a large baking dish, stir together the oil, shallots, salt, cumin, cinnamon, pepper, and chicken broth.
2. Add the chicken and sweet potatoes. Stir to coat with the spices. Place the dish in the preheated oven and bake for 35-45 minutes, or until the chicken is cooked through and the sweet potatoes are tender. Serve.

PER SERVING

Cal: 520; Fat 32g; Carbs 22g; Protein 32g

Slow Cooker Chicken Curry

Prep time: 5 minutes | Cook time: 4 hours 10 minutes | Serves 4

- 1½ lb chicken thighs
- 1 onion, sliced
- 2 garlic cloves, minced
- 1 tbsp coconut oil
- 1 tsp ground coriander
- 2 tsp ground cumin
- 1 tsp turmeric
- Sea salt and pepper to taste
- 1 (13-oz) can coconut milk
- 3 cups chicken broth
- ¼ cup chopped cilantro
- 2 scallions, sliced

1. Coat the slow cooker with coconut oil. Rub the chicken ground coriander, cumin, turmeric, salt, and pepper and add it to the slow cooker along with onion, garlic, coconut milk, and chicken broth.
2. Cover the slow cooker and cook on High for 4 hours. Garnish with the cilantro and scallions before serving.

PER SERVING

Cal: 650; Fat 55g; Carbs 10g; Protein 31g

Harissa Chicken Drumsticks

Prep time: 5 minutes | Cook time: 60 minutes + marinating time | Serves 4

- 2 garlic cloves, minced
- 1½ chicken drumsticks
- 1 cup coconut yogurt
- ½ cup extra-virgin olive oil
- Juice of 2 limes
- 1 tbsp raw honey
- Sea salt and pepper to taste
- 1 tsp ground cumin
- ½ tsp harissa seasoning
- ½ tsp turmeric

1. In a mixing bowl, whisk together the yogurt, olive oil, lime juice, garlic, honey, salt, cumin, harissa, turmeric, and pepper until smooth. Add the chicken and toss to coat. Cover with plastic wrap and chill for 30 minutes.
2. Discard the marinade. Place the sheet in the oven and bake the drumsticks for 25-35 minutes, or until they brown and are cooked through. Serve and enjoy!

PER SERVING

Cal: 375; Fat 30g; Carbs 9g; Protein 20g

Chicken Satay

Prep time: 5 minutes | Cook time: 25 minutes + marinating time | Serves 4

1 garlic clove, minced
½ cup peanut butter
2 tbsp coconut aminos
1 tbsp grated fresh ginger
3 tbsp lime juice
1 tsp raw honey
2 tsp sriracha sauce
1½ lb chicken breasts, cut into strips
2 tbsp olive oil
1 tbsp chopped cilantro

1. Combine the peanut butter, ¼ cup of water, coconut aminos, ginger, 1 tbsp of lime juice, garlic, and honey in your food processor and pulse until smooth. Set aside the sauce.
2. In a large bowl, whisk the remaining lime juice, cilantro, and sriracha sauce. Add the chicken strips and toss to coat. Cover the bowl with plastic wrap and refrigerate for 1 hour to marinate.
3. Preheat your oven to broil. Thread each chicken strip onto a wooden skewer and lay them on a rimmed baking sheet.
4. Broil the chicken for about 4 minutes per side until cooked through and golden, turning once. Serve with previously prepared sauce.

PER SERVING

Cal: 500; Fat 28g; Carbs 15g; Protein 45g

Herby Green Whole Chicken

Prep time: 5 minutes | Cook time: 1 hour 45 minutes | Serves 6

- 1 sweet onion, quartered
- 1 (4-lb) whole chicken
- 2 lemons, halved
- 4 garlic cloves, crushed
- 4 fresh thyme sprigs
- 4 fresh rosemary sprigs
- 4 fresh parsley sprigs
- 3 bay leaves
- 2 tbsp olive oil
- Sea salt and pepper to taste

1. Preheat your oven to 400°F. Put the chicken in a greased pan.
2. Stuff it with lemons, onion, garlic, thyme, rosemary, parsley, and bay leaves into the cavity. Brush the chicken with olive oil, and season lightly with sea salt and pepper.
3. Roast the chicken for about 1 ½ hours until golden brown and cooked through. Remove the chicken from the oven and let it sit for 10 minutes. Remove the lemons, onion, and herbs from the cavity and serve.

PER SERVING

Cal: 260; Fat 9g; Carbs 6g; Protein 39g

Chicken Thighs in Coconut Sauce

Prep time: 5 minutes | Cook time: 40 minutes | Serves 4

- 1 ½ cups canned coconut milk
- 1 sweet onion, quartered
- 2 tbsp grated fresh ginger
- Juice of 1 lime
- Zest of 1 lime
- 1 tbsp raw honey
- ½ tsp ground coriander
- 1 tbsp olive oil

1. Blend coconut milk, ginger, lime juice, lime zest, honey, and ground coriander in a bowl. Warm the olive oil in a skillet over medium heat.
2. Add the chicken thighs and sear for about 10 minutes or until golden, turning once. Pour the coconut milk mixture over the chicken and bring the liquid to a boil.
3. Reduce the heat to low, cover, and simmer for 15 minutes, or until the chicken is tender and cooked through. Serve garnished with scallions.

PER SERVING

Cal: 475; Fat 33g; Carbs 12g; Protein 34g

Homemade Chicken & Pepper Cacciatore

Prep time: 5 minutes | Cook time: 30 minutes | Serves 4

- 1 ½ lb chicken breasts, cubed
- 3 mixed peppers, cut into strips
- 28 oz canned diced tomatoes
- ½ cup chopped black olives
- 2 tbsp extra-virgin olive oil
- 1 tsp onion powder
- 1 tsp garlic powder
- Sea salt and pepper to taste

1. Warm the olive oil in a large saucepan over medium heat. Add the chicken and sauté for 8-10 minutes until evenly browned, stirring occasionally.
2. Add the peppers, tomatoes, olives, onion powder, garlic powder, salt, and pepper and allow to simmer for 10 minutes, stirring occasionally, or until the chicken is cooked through.

PER SERVING

Cal: 305; Fat 11g; Carbs 34g; Protein 18g

Broccoli & Chicken Stir-Fry

Prep time: 5 minutes | Cook time: 20 minutes | Serves 4

- 2 cups broccoli florets
- 1 ½ lb chicken breasts, cubed
- ½ onion, chopped
- Sea salt and pepper to taste
- 3 tbsp extra-virgin olive oil
- 3 garlic cloves, minced

1. Warm the olive oil in a skillet over medium heat.
2. Add the broccoli, chicken, garlic, and onion and stir-fry for about 8 minutes, or until the chicken is golden browned and cooked through. Season with salt and pepper. Serve.

PER SERVING

Cal: 345; Fat 13g; Carbs 4g; Protein 13g

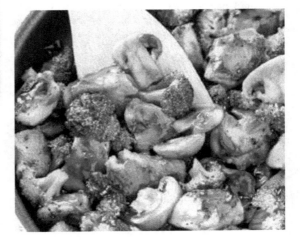

Sicilian Chicken Bake

Prep time: 5 minutes | Cook time: 30 minutes | Serves 4

- 1 cup sliced cremini mushrooms
- 4 garlic cloves, minced
- 4 chicken breasts
- 2 tbsp avocado oil
- 1 cup chopped spinach
- 1 fennel bulb, sliced
- 20 cherry tomatoes, halved
- ½ cup chopped fresh basil
- ½ red onion, thinly sliced
- 2 tsp balsamic vinegar

1. Preheat your oven to 400°F. Arrange the chicken breasts on a baking dish and brush them generously with avocado oil.
2. Mix together the mushrooms, spinach, fennel, tomatoes, basil, red onion, garlic, and balsamic vinegar in a medium bowl and toss to combine. Top the breasts with the vegetable mixture.
3. Bake in the oven for about 20 minutes, or until the juices run clear when pierced with a fork. Allow the chicken to rest for 5-10 minutes before slicing. Serve and enjoy!

PER SERVING

Cal: 225; Fat 8g; Carbs 7g; Protein 27g

Chicken a la Tuscana

Prep time: 5 minutes | Cook time: 25 minutes | Serves 4

- 2 cups cherry tomatoes
- 4 chicken breast halves
- 1 tsp garlic powder
- Sea salt and pepper to taste
- 2 tbsp extra-virgin olive oil
- ½ cup sliced green olives
- 1 eggplant, chopped
- ¼ cup dry white wine

1. Pound the chicken breasts with a meat tenderizer until half an inch thick. Rub them with garlic powder, salt, and ground black pepper. Warm the olive oil in a skillet over medium heat.
2. Add the chicken and cook for 14-16 minutes, flipping halfway through the cooking time. Transfer to a plate and cover with aluminum foil.
3. Add the tomatoes, olives, and eggplant to the skillet and sauté for 4 minutes or until the vegetables are soft.
4. Add the white wine to the skillet and simmer for 1 minute. Remove the aluminum foil and top the chicken with the vegetables and their juices, then serve warm.

PER SERVING

Cal: 170; Fat 10g; Carbs 8g; Protein 7g

Baked Basil Chicken

Prep time: 5 minutes | Cook time: 45 minutes | Serves 4

- 2 garlic cloves, sliced
- 1 white onion, chopped
- 14 oz tomatoes, chopped
- 2 tbsp chopped rosemary
- Sea salt and pepper to taste
- 4 skinless chicken thighs
- 1 lb peeled pumpkin, cubed
- 1 tbsp extra virgin olive oil
- 2 tbsp basil leaves

1. Preheat your oven to 375°F. Warm the olive oil in a skillet over medium heat. Add the garlic and onion and sauté for 5 minutes or until fragrant.
2. Add the tomatoes, rosemary, salt, and pepper and cook for 15 minutes or until slightly thickened. Arrange the chicken thighs and pumpkin cubes on a baking sheet, then pour the mixture in the skillet over the chicken and sweet potatoes.
3. Stir to coat well. Pour in enough water to cover the chicken and sweet potatoes. Bake in for 20 minutes. Top with basil.

PER SERVING

Cal: 295; Fat 9g; Carbs 32g; Protein 21g

Mumbai-Inspired Chicken

Prep time: 5 minutes | Cook time: 30 minutes | Serves 6

- 2 chicken breasts, cubed
- 2 carrots, diced
- 1 white onion, diced
- 1 tbsp minced fresh ginger
- 6 garlic cloves, minced
- 1 cup sugar snap peas, diced
- 1 (5-oz) can coconut cream
- 2 tbsp coconut oil, divided
- cup diced tomatoes
- ½ tsp garam masala
- Sea salt and pepper to taste
- ¼ tsp cayenne pepper

1. Warm the coconut oil in a skillet over medium. Add the chicken breasts and cook for 15 minutes, stirring occasionally; reserve.
2. Add the carrots, onion, ginger, and garlic to the same skillet and sauté for 5 minutes or until fragrant and the onion is translucent.
3. Add the peas, coconut cream, fish sauce, chicken broth, tomatoes, garam masala, salt, cayenne pepper, pepper, and ¼ cup of water. Stir. Bring to a boil. Reduce the heat and simmer for 10 minutes. return the cooked chicken and cook for 2 more minutes. Serve immediately.

PER SERVING

Cal: 220; Fat 15g; Carbs 9g; Protein 13g

Jerk Chicken Drumsticks

Prep time: 5 minutes | Cook time: 4 hours 15 minutes | Serves 4

- 1 lb chicken drumsticks
- ¼ cup cilantro, chopped
- 3 tbsp lime juice
- ½ tsp garlic powder
- ½ tsp sea salt
- 1 tbsp jerk seasoning

1. In a small bowl, stir together the cilantro, lime juice, garlic powder, salt, and jerk seasoning to form a paste.
2. Put the drumsticks in your slow cooker. Spread the cilantro paste evenly on each drumstick.
3. Cover the cooker and set to "High". Cook for 4 hours, or until the juices run clear. Leave to rest for 10 minutes. Serve and enjoy!

PER SERVING

Cal: 415; Fat 11g; Carbs 1g; Protein 70g

Oregano Braised Chicken Legs

Prep time: 5 minutes | Cook time: 8 hours 15 minutes | Serves 4

- 1 lb chicken legs
- 1 onion, thickly sliced
- 1 tsp garlic powder
- 1 tsp chili powder
- 1 tsp paprika
- 1 tsp dried oregano
- Sea salt and pepper to taste

1. In a mixing bowl, stir together the garlic powder, chili powder, paprika, oregano, salt, and pepper.
2. Rub the spice mix all over the chicken legs. Place them in your slow cooker along with the sliced onion.
3. Cover the cooker and set to "Low". Cook for 6-8 hours, or until very tender. Rest for 15 minutes before carving. Serve and enjoy!

PER SERVING

Cal: 860; Fat 58g; Carbs 7g; Protein 85g

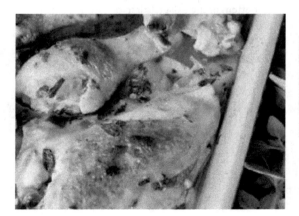

The Best General Tso's Chicken

Prep time: 5 minutes | Cook time: 30 minutes | Serves 4

- 3 tbsp coconut aminos
- 1 tsp Shaoxing wine
- 1 tbsp arrowroot powder
- ½ tsp red pepper flakes
- 2 garlic cloves, minced
- 2 tbsp rice vinegar
- 3 tbsp coconut sugar
- ¼ tsp ground ginger
- 1 tbsp almond butter
- 1 lb chicken breasts, cubed
- 1 tbsp avocado oil
- 1 cup brown rice flour
- ¼ tsp garlic powder
- ¼ tsp sea salt

1. Cook the ginger and almond butter in a saucepan over medium heat for 2 minutes.
2. Add the coconut aminos, Shaoxing wine, arrowroot powder, red pepper flakes, garlic, vinegar, and coconut sugar to the saucepan. Stir to mix well. Bring to a boil. Reduce the heat t and simmer for 5 minutes or until the sauce is thickened.
3. Heat the avocado oil in a nonstick skillet over medium heat. Combine the rice flour, garlic powder, and sea salt in a small bowl. Mix well.
4. Dip the chicken in the mixture, then place in the skillet and cook for 8 minutes or until golden brown and crispy. Flip the chicken halfway through the cooking time. Transfer the chicken thighs to a large plate and pour over it the sauce. Serve and enjoy!

PER SERVING

Cal: 480; Fat 20g; Carbs 41g; Protein 32g

Moroccan-Style Chicken Thighs

Prep time: 5 minutes | Cook time: 8 hours 15 minutes | Serves 4

- 2 lb boneless, skinless chicken thighs
- 2 cups chicken broth
- 8 green olives, sliced
- 1 tsp sea salt
- Juice and zest of 1 lemon

1. In a bowl, stir together the salt, lemon juice, and lemon zest. Coat the chicken thighs with the mixture.
2. Pour the broth and olives into your slow cooker. Add the thighs to the slow cooker.
3. Cover the cooker and set to "Low". Cook for 7-8 hours, or until tender and cooked through. Serve and enjoy!

PER SERVING

Cal: 285; Fat 13g; Carbs 3g; Protein 42g

Turmeric Chicken & Chickpea Stew

Prep time: 5 minutes | Cook time: 4 hours 15 minutes | Serves 4

- 1 lb boneless, skinless chicken thighs
- 1 onion, thinly sliced
- 2 garlic cloves, thinly sliced
- 1 tbsp extra-virgin olive oil
- 1 tsp minced ginger root
- 2 tsp ground turmeric
- 1 tsp fennel seeds, crushed
- Sea salt and pepper to taste
- 2 cups chicken broth
- 1 cup coconut milk
- ¼ cup chopped cilantro

1. Grease your slow cooker with olive oil.
2. Add the chicken, onion, garlic, ginger root, turmeric, fennel seeds, salt, pepper, chicken broth, and coconut milk, and toss to combine.
3. Cover and cook on "High" for 4 hours. Garnish with the chopped cilantro and serve.

PER SERVING

Cal: 375; Fat 18g; Carbs 4g; Protein 45g

Korean Chicken Thighs

Prep time: 5 minutes | Cook time: 4 hours 10 minutes | Serves 4

- 8 boneless, skinless chicken thighs
- ¼ cup miso paste
- 2 tbsp coconut oil, melted
- 1 tbsp honey
- 1 tbsp rice wine vinegar
- 2 garlic cloves, sliced
- 1 tsp minced ginger root
- 2 red chilies, sliced
- 1 cup chicken broth
- 2 scallions, sliced
- 1 tbsp sesame seeds

1. Place the miso, coconut oil, honey, rice wine vinegar, garlic, chilies, and ginger root in your slow cooker and mix well.
2. Add the chicken. Cover and cook on "High" for 4 hours. Top with scallions and sesame seeds. Serve.

PER SERVING

Cal: 315; Fat 14g; Carbs 17g; Protein 31g

Pan-Fried Turkey Meatballs

Prep time: 5 minutes | Cook time: 20 minutes | Serves 4

- 2 tbsp sesame oil
- ½ tsp ground cumin
- 1½ lb ground turkey
- 1 cup shredded cabbage
- ¼ cup chopped cilantro
- 1 tbsp grated fresh ginger
- 1 tsp garlic powder
- 1 tsp onion powder
- Sea salt and pepper to taste

1. Mix the turkey, cumin, cabbage, cilantro, ginger, garlic powder, onion powder, salt, and pepper in a bowl. Roll the mixture into about 18-20 balls.
2. Warm the sesame oil in a skillet over medium heat. Once hot, sear the meatballs in the pan until browned on all sides, 10 minutes. Serve.

PER SERVING

Cal 410; Fat 27g; Carbs 5g; Protein 2g

Lemon & Caper Turkey Scaloppine

Prep time: 5 minutes | Cook time: 25 minutes | Serves 4

- 1 tbsp capers
- ¼ cup whole-wheat flour
- Sea salt and pepper to taste
- 4 turkey breast cutlets
- 2 tbsp olive oil
- 3 lemons, juiced
- 1 lemon, zested
- 1 tbsp chopped parsley

1. Pound the turkey with a rolling pin to ¼-inch thickness. Combine flour, salt, and pepper in a bowl. Roll each cutlet piece in the flour, shaking off the excess.
2. Warm the olive oil in a skillet over medium heat. Sear the cutlets for 4 minutes on both sides. Transfer to a plate and cover with aluminium foil.
3. Pour the lemon juice and lemon zest in the skillet to scrape up the browned bits that stick to the bottom of the skillet. Stir in capers and rosemary. Cook for 2 minutes until the sauce has thickened slightly. Drizzle the sauce over the cutlets. Serve.

PER SERVING

Cal 190; Fat 14g; Carbs 9g; Protein 2g3

Ground Turkey & Spinach Stir-Fry

Prep time: 5 minutes | Cook time: 20 minutes | Serves 4

- 2 tbsp olive oil
- 1 ½ lb ground turkey
- 2 cups chopped spinach
- 4 green onions, sliced
- 2 tbsp fresh thyme
- Sea salt and pepper to taste
- 2 garlic cloves, minced

1. Warm the olive oil in a skillet over medium heat. Brown the turkey, breaking apart with a wide spatula for about 6 minutes.
2. Add the spinach, green onions, garlic, thyme, salt, and pepper. Cook for 3-5 minutes, stirring often.

PER SERVING

Cal 420; Fat 21g; Carbs 8g; Protein 2g

Chicken Bone Broth

Prep time: 15 minutes or fewer | Cook time: 6 to 8 hours on low | Makes

- about 12 cups
- 1 chicken carcass
- About 12 cups filtered water (enough to cover the bones)
- 2 carrots, roughly chopped
- 2 garlic cloves, roughly chopped
- 1 celery stalk, roughly chopped
- ½ onion, roughly chopped
- 2 bay leaves
- 1 parsley sprig
- ¾ teaspoon sea salt
- ½ teaspoon dried oregano
- ½ teaspoon dried basil leaves
- 1 tablespoon apple cider vinegar

1. In your slow cooker, combine the chicken carcass, water, carrots, garlic, celery, onion, bay leaves, parsley, salt, oregano, basil, and vinegar.
2. Cover the cooker and set to low. Cook for 6 to 8 hours.
3. Skim off any scum from the surface of the broth, and pour the broth through a fine-mesh sieve into a large bowl, discarding the chicken and veggie scraps. Refrigerate the broth in an airtight container for up to 5 days, or freeze it for up to 3 months.

PER SERVING

Calories: 50; Total Fat: 1g; Total Carbs: 1g; Sugar: 0g; Fiber: 0g; Protein: 9g; Sodium: 145mg

Basic "Rotisserie" Chicken

Prep time: 15 minutes or fewer | Cook time: 6 to 8 hours on low | Serves 4

- 1 teaspoon garlic powder
- 1 teaspoon chili powder
- 1 teaspoon paprika
- 1 teaspoon dried thyme leaves
- 1 teaspoon sea salt
- Pinch cayenne pepper
- Freshly ground black pepper
- 1 whole chicken (about 4 to 5 pounds), neck and giblets removed
- ½ medium onion, sliced

1. In a small bowl, stir together the garlic powder, chili powder, paprika, thyme, salt, and cayenne. Season with black pepper, and stir again to combine. Rub the spice mix all over the exterior of the chicken.
2. Place the chicken in the slow cooker with the sliced onion sprinkled around it.
3. Cover the cooker and set to low. Cook for 6 to 8 hours, or until the internal temperature reaches 165°F on a meat thermometer and the juices run clear, and serve.

PER SERVING

Calories: 862; Total Fat: 59g; Total Carbs: 7g; Sugar: 6g; Fiber: 0g; Protein: 86g; Sodium: 1,200mg

Tangy Barbecue Chicken

Prep time: 15 minutes or fewer | Cook time: 3 to 4 hours on high | Serves 4

- 4 to 5 boneless, skinless chicken breasts (about 2 pounds)
- 2 cups tangy barbecue sauce with apple cider vinegar

1. In your slow cooker, combine the chicken and barbecue sauce. Stir until the chicken breasts are well coated in the sauce.
2. Cover the cooker and set to high. Cook for 3 to 4 hours, or until the internal temperature of the chicken reaches 165°F on a meat thermometer and the juices run clear.
3. Shred the chicken with a fork, mix it into the sauce, and serve.

PER SERVING

Calories: 412; Total Fat: 13g; Total Carbs: 22g; Sugar: 19g; Fiber: 0g; Protein: 51g; Sodium: 766mg

Salsa Verde Chicken

Prep time: 15 minutes or fewer| Cook time:6 to 8 hours on low | Serves 4

- 4 to 5 boneless, skinless chicken breasts (about 2 pounds)
- 2 cups green salsa
- 1 cup chicken broth
- 2 tablespoons freshly squeezed lime juice
- 1 teaspoon sea salt
- 1 teaspoon chili powder

1. In your slow cooker, combine the chicken, salsa, broth, lime juice, salt, and chili powder. Stir to combine.
2. Cover the cooker and set to low. Cook for 6 to 8 hours, or until the internal temperature of the chicken reaches 165°F on a meat thermometer and the juices run clear.
3. Shred the chicken with a fork, mix it into the sauce, and serve.

PER SERVING

Calories: 318; Total Fat: 8g; Total Carbs: 6g; Sugar: 2g; Fiber: 1g; Protein: 52g; Sodium: 1,510mg

Lemon & Garlic Chicken Thighs

Prep time: 15 minutes or fewer| Cook time:7 to 8 hours on low | Serves 4

- 2 cups chicken broth
- 1½ teaspoons garlic powder
- 1 teaspoon sea salt
- Juice and zest of 1 large lemon
- 2 pounds boneless skinless chicken thighs

1. Pour the broth into the slow cooker.
2. In a small bowl, stir together the garlic powder, salt, lemon juice, and lemon zest. Baste each chicken thigh with an even coating of the mixture. Place the thighs along the bottom of the slow cooker.
3. Cover the cooker and set to low. Cook for 7 to 8 hours, or until the internal temperature of the chicken reaches 165°F on a meat thermometer and the juices run clear, and serve.

PER SERVING

Calories: 290; Total Fat: 14g; Total Carbs: 3g; Sugar: 0g; Fiber: 0g; Protein: 43g; Sodium: 1,017mg

Slow Cooker Chicken Fajitas

Prep time: 15 minutes or fewer| Cook time:7 to 8 hours on low | Serves 4

- 1 (14.5-ounce) can diced tomatoes
- 1 (4-ounce) can Hatch green chiles
- 1½ teaspoons garlic powder
- 2 teaspoons chili powder
- 1½ teaspoons ground cumin
- 1 teaspoon paprika
- 1 teaspoon sea salt
- Juice of 1 lime
- Pinch cayenne pepper
- Freshly ground black pepper
- 1 red bell pepper, seeded and sliced
- 1 green bell pepper, seeded and sliced
- 1 yellow bell pepper, seeded and sliced
- 1 large onion, sliced
- 2 pounds boneless, skinless chicken breast

1. In a medium bowl, combine the diced tomatoes, chiles, garlic powder, chili powder, cumin, paprika, salt, lime juice, and cayenne, and season with black pepper. Mix well. Pour half the diced tomato mixture into the bottom of your slow cooker.
2. Layer half the red, green, and yellow bell peppers and half the onion over the tomatoes in the cooker.
3. Place the chicken on top of the peppers and onions.
4. Cover the chicken with the remaining red, green, and yellow bell peppers and onions. Pour the remaining tomato mixture on top.
5. Cover the cooker and set to low. Cook for 7 to 8 hours, or until the internal temperature of the chicken reaches 165°F on a meat thermometer and the juices run clear, and serve.

PER SERVING

Calories: 310; Total Fat: 5g; Total Carbs: 19g; Sugar: 7g; Fiber: 4g; Protein: 46g; Sodium: 1,541mg

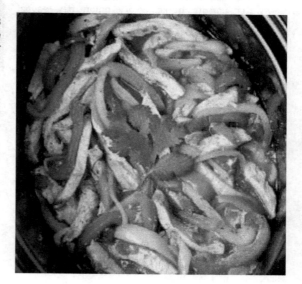

White Bean, Chicken & Apple Cider Chili

Prep time: 15 minutes or fewer| Cook time:7 to 8 hours on low | Serves 4

- 3 cups chopped cooked chicken
- 2 (15-ounce) cans white navy beans, rinsed well and drained
- 1 medium onion, chopped
- 1 (15-ounce) can diced tomatoes
- 3 cups Chicken Bone Broth or store-bought chicken broth
- 1 cup apple cider
- 2 bay leaves
- 1 tablespoon extra-virgin olive oil
- 2 teaspoons garlic powder
- 1 teaspoon chili powder
- 1 teaspoon sea salt
- ½ teaspoon ground cumin
- ¼ teaspoon ground cinnamon
- Pinch cayenne pepper
- Freshly ground black pepper
- ¼ cup apple cider vinegar

1. In your slow cooker, combine the chicken, beans, onion, tomatoes, broth, cider, bay leaves, olive oil, garlic powder, chili powder, salt, cumin, cinnamon, and cayenne, and season with black pepper.
2. Cover the cooker and set to low. Cook for 7 to 8 hours.
3. Remove and discard the bay leaves. Stir in the apple cider vinegar until well blended and serve.

PER SERVING

Calories: 469; Total Fat: 8g; Total Carbs: 46g; Sugar: 13g; Fiber: 9g; Protein: 51g; Sodium: 1,047mg

Buffalo Chicken Lettuce Wraps

Prep time: 15 minutes or fewer| Cook time:7 to 8 hours on low | Serves 4

- 1 tablespoon extra-virgin olive oil
- 2 pounds boneless, skinless chicken breast
- 2 cups vegan buffalo dip
- 1 cup water
- 8 to 10 romaine lettuce leaves
- ½ red onion, thinly sliced
- 1 cup cherry tomatoes, halved

1. Coat the bottom of the slow cooker with the olive oil.
2. Cover the cooker and set to low. Cook for 7 to 8 hours, or until the internal temperature of the chicken reaches 165°F on a meat thermometer and the juices run clear.
3. Shred the chicken with a fork, and mix it into the dip in the slow cooker.
4. Divide the meat mixture among the lettuce leaves. Top with onion and tomato, and serve.

PER SERVING

Calories: 437; Total Fat: 18g; Total Carbs: 18g; Sugar: 8g; Fiber: 4g; Protein: 49g; Sodium: 993mg

Cilantro-Lime Chicken Drumsticks

Prep time: 15 minutes or fewer| Cook time:2 to 3 hours on high | Serves 4

- ¼ cup fresh cilantro, chopped
- 3 tablespoons freshly squeezed lime juice
- ½ teaspoon garlic powder
- ½ teaspoon sea salt
- ¼ teaspoon ground cumin
- 3 pounds chicken drumsticks

1. In a small bowl, stir together the cilantro, lime juice, garlic powder, salt, and cumin to form a paste.
2. Put the drumsticks in the slow cooker. Spread the cilantro paste evenly on each drumstick.
3. Cover the cooker and set to high. Cook for 2 to 3 hours, or until the internal temperature of the chicken reaches 165°F on a meat thermometer and the juices run clear, and serve.

PER SERVING

Calories: 417; Total Fat: 12g; Total Carbs: 1g; Sugar: 1g; Fiber: 1g; Protein: 71g; Sodium: 591mg

Coconut-Curry-Cashew Chicken

Prep time: 15 minutes or fewer| Cook time:7 to 8 hours on low | Serves 4

- 1½ cups chicken bone broth
- 1 (14-ounce) can full-fat coconut milk
- 1 teaspoon garlic powder
- 1 tablespoon red curry paste
- 1 teaspoon sea salt
- ½ teaspoon freshly ground black pepper
- ½ teaspoon coconut sugar
- 2 pounds boneless, skinless chicken breasts
- 1½ cup unsalted cashews
- ½ cup diced white onion

1. In a medium bowl, combine the broth, coconut milk, garlic powder, red curry paste, salt, pepper, and coconut sugar. Stir well.
2. Put the chicken, cashews, and onion in the slow cooker. Pour the coconut milk, mixture on top.
3. Cover the cooker and set to low. Cook for 7 to 8 hours, or until the internal temperature of the chicken reaches 165°F on a meat thermometer and the juices run clear.
4. Shred the chicken with a fork, and mix it into the cooking liquid. You can also remove the chicken from the broth and chop it with a knife into bite-size pieces before returning it to the slow cooker. Serve.

PER SERVING

Calories: 714; Total Fat: 43g; Total Carbs: 21g; Sugar: 5g; Fiber: 3g; Protein: 57g; Sodium: 1,606mg

Sesame Miso Chicken

Prep Time: 10 minutes | Cook time: 4 Hours| Serves 4

- ¼ cup white miso
- 2 tablespoons coconut oil, melted
- 2 tablespoons honey
- 1 tablespoon unseasoned rice wine vinegar
- 2 garlic cloves, thinly sliced
- 1 teaspoon minced fresh ginger root
- 1 cup chicken broth
- 8 boneless, skinless chicken thighs
- 2 scallions, sliced
- 1 tablespoon sesame seeds

1. In a slow cooker, combine the miso, coconut oil, honey, rice wine vinegar, garlic, and ginger root, mixing well.
2. Add the chicken and toss to combine. Cover and cook on high for 4 hours.
3. Transfer the chicken and sauce to a serving dish. Garnish with the scallions and sesame seeds and serve.

PER SERVING

Calories: 320; Total Fat: 15g; Total Carbohydrates: 17g; Sugar: 11g; Fiber: 1g; Protein: 32g; Sodium: 1,020mg

Ginger Turkey Burgers

Prep Time: 10 minutes | Cook time: 10 minutes| Serves 4

- 1½ pounds ground turkey
- 1 large egg, lightly beaten
- 2 tablespoons coconut flour (or almond flour)
- ½ cup finely chopped onion
- 1 garlic clove, minced
- 2 teaspoons minced fresh ginger root
- 1 tablespoon fresh cilantro
- 1 teaspoon salt
- ¼ teaspoon freshly ground black pepper
- 1 tablespoon extra-virgin olive oil

1. In a medium bowl, combine the ground turkey, egg, flour, onion, garlic, ginger root, cilantro, salt, and pepper and mix well.
2. Form the turkey mixture into four patties.
3. Heat the olive oil in a large skillet over medium-high heat.
4. Cook the burgers, flipping once, until firm to the touch, 3 to 4 minutes on each side. Serve.

PER SERVING

Calories: 320; Total Fat: 20g; Total Carbohydrates: 2g; Sugar: 1g; Fiber: <1g; Protein: 34g; Sodium: 720mg

Mushroom Turkey Thighs

Prep Time: 15 minutes | Cook time: 4 Hours| Serves 4

- 1 tablespoon extra-virgin olive oil
- 2 turkey thighs
- 2 cups button or cremini mushrooms, sliced
- 1 large onion, sliced
- 1 garlic clove, sliced
- 1 rosemary sprig
- 1 teaspoon salt
- ¼ teaspoon freshly ground black pepper
- 2 cups chicken broth
- ½ cup dry red wine

1. Drizzle the olive oil into a slow cooker. Add the turkey thighs, mushrooms, onion, garlic, rosemary sprig, salt, and pepper. Pour in the chicken broth and wine. Cover and cook on high for 4 hours.
2. Remove and discard the rosemary sprig. Use a slotted spoon to transfer the thighs to a plate and allow them to cool for several minutes for easier handling.
3. Cut the meat from the bones, stir the meat into the mushrooms, and serve.

PER SERVING

Calories: 280; Total Fat: 9g; Total Carbohydrates: 3g; Sugar: 1g; Fiber: <1g; Protein: 43g; Sodium: 850mg

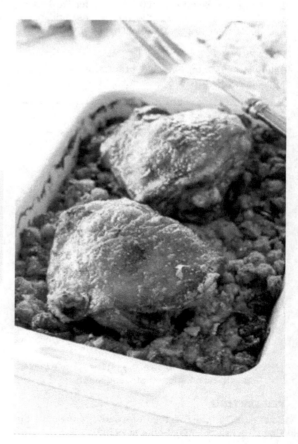

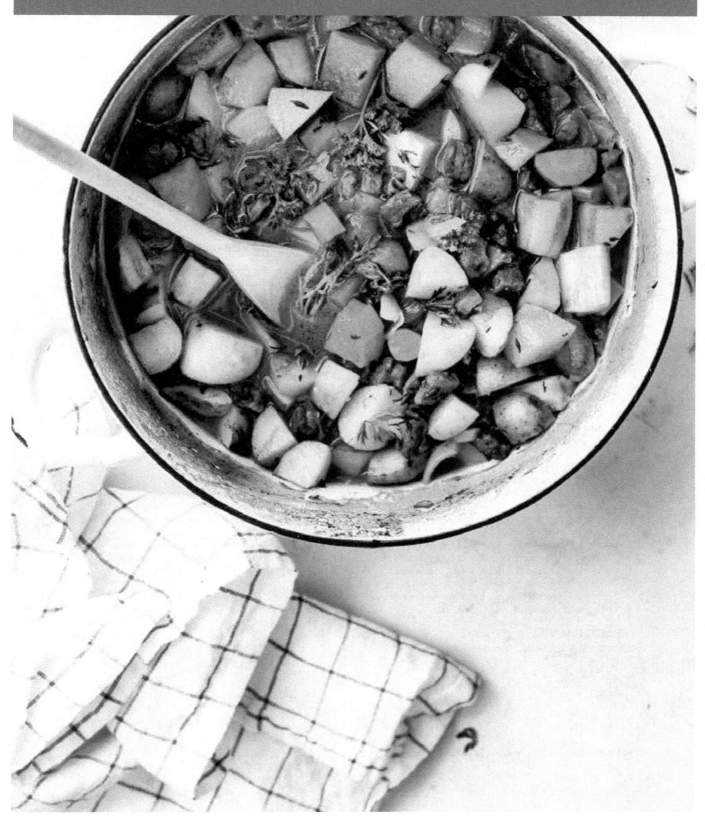

Chapter 8
Meat Dishes

Beef Meatloaf with Horseradish

Prep time: 5 minutes | Cook time: 70 minutes | Serves 4

- ½ cup almond flour
- ½ cup chopped sweet onion
- 1½ lb ground beef
- 1 egg
- 1 tbsp chopped fresh basil
- 1 tsp Dijon mustard
- 1 tsp grated horseradish
- ⅛ tsp sea salt

1. Preheat your oven to 350°F.
2. In a mixing bowl, combine the ground beef, almond flour, onion, egg, basil, mustard, horseradish, and sea salt until well mixed.
3. Press the meatloaf mixture into a loaf pan. Bake for about 1 hour until cooked through. Remove the meatloaf from the oven and let it rest for 10 minutes before slicing.

PER SERVING

Cal 405; Fat 17g; Carbs 4g; Protein 55g

Herbed Lamb Roast with Sweet Potatoes

Prep time: 5 minutes | Cook time: 70 minutes | Serves 4

- 1 (3-lb) lamb leg
- 1 tsp dried sage
- 1 tsp dried marjoram
- 1 bay leaf, crushed
- 1 tsp dried thyme
- 3 garlic cloves, minced
- 1 lb sweet potatoes, cubed
- 2 tbsp olive oil
- 3 tbsp arrowroot powder
- 2 cups chicken broth
- Sea salt and pepper to taste

1. Heat the oil in your Instant Pot on "Sauté". Combine the herbs with some salt and pepper and rub the mixture into the meat. Brown the lamb on all sides.
2. Pour the broth around the meat, close the lid, and cook for 60 minutes on "Manual".
3. Release the pressure quickly and add the potatoes. Close the lid and cook for 10 more minutes. Transfer the meat and potatoes to a plate.
4. Combine 1 cup of water and arrowroot and stir the mixture into the pot sauce. Pour the gravy over the meat and potatoes.

PER SERVING

Cal 740; Fat 57g; Carbs 1g; Protein 57g

Saucy Tomato Beef Meatballs

Prep time: 5 minutes | Cook time: 8 hours 15 minutes | Serves 6

- 1½ lb ground beef
- 1 can crushed tomatoes
- 1 large egg
- 1 small onion, minced
- ¼ cup minced mushrooms
- 1 tsp garlic powder
- Sea salt and pepper to taste
- ½ tsp dried thyme
- ¼ tsp ground ginger
- ¼ tsp red pepper flakes

1. Combine the ground beef, egg, onion, mushrooms, garlic powder, salt, pepper, thyme, ginger, and red pepper flakes in a large bowl. Mix well.
2. Form the beef mixture into about 12 meatballs. Pour the tomatoes into your slow cooker. Gently arrange the meatballs on top.
3. Cover the cooker and set to "Low". Cook for 8 hours.

PER SERVING

Cal 130; Fat 9g; Carbs 2g; Protein 10g

Traditional Beef Bolognese

Prep time: 5 minutes | Cook time: 8 hours 15 minutes | Serves 4

- 3 garlic cloves, minced
- 1 tbsp extra-virgin olive oil
- 1 chopped onion
- 1 chopped celery stalk
- 1 chopped carrot
- 1 lb ground beef
- 1 can diced tomatoes
- 1 tbsp white wine vinegar
- ⅛ tsp ground nutmeg
- ½ cup red wine
- ½ tsp red pepper flakes
- Sea salt and pepper to taste

1. Grease your slow cooker with olive oil.
2. Add onion, garlic, celery, carrot, ground beef, tomatoes, vinegar, nutmeg, wine, pepper flakes, salt, and pepper.
3. Using a fork, break up the ground beef as much as possible. Cover the cooker and cook for 8 hours on "Low". Serve and enjoy!

PER SERVING

Cal 315; Fat 20g; Carbs 10g; Protein 21g

Lettuce-Wrapped Beef Roast

Prep time: 5 minutes | Cook time: 8 hours 15 minutes | Serves 4

- 2 lb beef chuck roast
- 1 shallot, diced
- 1 cup beef broth
- 3 tbsp coconut aminos
- 1 tbsp rice vinegar
- 1 tsp garlic powder
- 1 tsp olive oil
- ½ tsp ground ginger
- ¼ tsp red pepper flakes
- 8 romaine lettuce leaves
- 1 tbsp sesame seeds
- 1 scallion, diced

1. Place the beef, shallot, broth, coconut aminos, vinegar, garlic powder, olive oil, ginger, and red pepper flakes in your slow cooker.
2. Cover the cooker and set to "Low". Cook for 8 hours. Scoop spoonfuls of the beef mixture into each lettuce leaf. Top with sesame seeds and scallion.

PER SERVING

Cal 425; Fat 22g; Carbs 12g; Protein 45g

Rosemary Lamb Chops

Prep time: 5 minutes | Cook time: 50 minutes + marinating time | Serves 4

- 4 garlic cloves, mashed
- 8 lamb chops
- 2 tbsp chopped rosemary
- ¼ cup extra-virgin olive oil
- 1 tsp Dijon mustard
- Sea salt and pepper to taste

1. Mix the olive oil, rosemary, garlic, Dijon mustard, salt, and pepper in a bowl. Add the lamb chops and toss to coat R.
2. Cover the dish with plastic wrap and marinate the chops at room temperature for 30 minutes. Preheat your oven to 425°F.
3. Bake the lamb chops for 15-20 minutes, or until they are sizzling and browned. Serve.

PER SERVING

Cal 645; Fat 33g; Carbs 3g; Protein 79g

Mustardy Leg of Lamb

Prep time: 5 minutes | Cook time: 6 hours 15 minutes | Serves 4

- 1 (3-lb) lamb leg
- ½ cup white wine
- 1½ cups chicken broth
- 1 onion, roughly chopped
- Sea salt and pepper to taste
- 1 tsp garlic powder
- 1 tsp dried rosemary
- 1 tsp Dijon mustard

1. Make a paste in a small bowl by stirring together mustard, garlic powder, rosemary, salt, and pepper.
2. Rub the paste evenly onto the lamb and put it in your slow cooker. Pour in broth, white wine, and onion around the lamb. Cover with the lid and cook for 6 hours on "Low". Serve.

PER SERVING

Cal 780; Fat 40g; Carbs 3g; Protein 92g

Tomato & Lentil Lamb Ragù

Prep time: 5 minutes | Cook time: 40 minutes | Serves 4

- 1 red onion, chopped
- 4 garlic cloves, minced
- 1 lb ground lamb
- 14 oz canned diced tomatoes
- 1 cup chicken broth
- 2 tbsp extra-virgin olive oil
- ½ cup green lentils
- Sea salt and pepper to taste
- 1 tsp ginger powder
- 1 tsp ground cumin

1. Warm the olive oil in a large pan over high heat. Add the onion and garlic sauté for 3 minutes.
2. Add the ground lamb, breaking it up with a spoon. Brown for 3-4 minutes. Stir in the tomatoes, chicken broth, lentils, salt, ginger powder, cumin, and pepper.
3. Simmer for 20 minutes, or until the lentils are cooked and most of the liquid has evaporated. Serve and enjoy!

PER SERVING

Cal 400; Fat 15g; Carbs 23g; Protein 40g

Smoky Lamb Souvlaki

Prep time: 5 minutes | Cook time: 25 minutes + marinating time | Serves 4

- 1 lb lamb shoulder, cubed
- 2 tbsp olive oil
- 1 tbsp apple cider vinegar
- 2 tsp crushed fennel seeds
- 2 tsp smoked paprika
- Salt and garlic powder to taste

1. Blend the olive oil, cider vinegar, crushed fennel seeds, smoked paprika, garlic powder, and sea salt in a large bowl. Stir in the lamb.
2. Cover the bowl and refrigerate it for 1 hour to marinate. Preheat a frying pan over high heat. Thread 4-5 pieces of lamb each onto 8 skewers. Fry for 3-4 minutes per side until cooked through. Serve.

PER SERVING

Cal 275; Fat 15g; Carbs 1g; Protein 31g

Pork Tenderloin with Garlic & Herbs

Prep time: 5 minutes | Cook time: 30 minutes | Serves 4

- ½ cup fresh parsley
- ¼ cup Dijon mustard
- 6 garlic cloves
- 2 tbsp fresh thyme
- 2 tbsp fresh cilantro
- 1 lime, zested
- 3 tbsp olive oil
- Sea salt and pepper to taste
- 1½-lb pork tenderloin

1. Preheat your oven to 400°F. Place parsley, mustard, garlic, cilantro, thyme, lime zest, olive oil, salt, and pepper in a food processor. Process for 20 seconds until it reaches a paste consistency.
2. Brush the tenderloin with the paste and place it on a parchment-lined baking sheet. Bake for 15 minutes until the meat reaches an internal temperature of 160°F. Let it sit for 5 minutes before slicing. Serve.

PER SERVING

Cal 370; Fat 19g; Carbs 6g; Protein 3g

Apple-Ginger Pork Chops

Prep time: 5 minutes | Cook time: 25 minutes | Serves 4

- 4 thin-cut pork chops
- Sea salt and pepper to taste
- 6 cored apples, chopped
- ¼ tsp ground allspice
- ¼ cup raw honey
- 1 tbsp grated fresh ginger

1. Preheat your oven to 425°F. Sprinkle pork chops with salt and pepper. Place the chops on a lined baking sheet and bake for 15 minutes until the meat is cooked.
2. Place the apples, allspice, brown sugar, ¼ cup of water, and ginger in a pot over medium heat and cook covered for 10 minutes until the apples are tender and thoroughly cooked.
3. Pour the sauce over the chops and serve warm.

PER SERVING

Cal 450; Fat 11g; Carbs 57g; Protein 9g

Mustard Pork Chops with Collard Greens

Prep time: 5 minutes | Cook time: 25 minutes | Serves 4

- 4 thin-cut pork chops
- Sea salt and pepper to taste
- 4 tbsp Dijon mustard
- 3 tbsp olive oil
- ½ red onion, finely chopped
- 4 cups chopped collard greens
- 2 tbsp apple cider vinegar

1. Preheat your oven to 425°F. Sprinkle pork chops with salt and pepper. Rub them with 2 tbsp of mustard and transfer to a parchment-lined baking sheet. Bake for 15 minutes until the pork is cooked through.
2. Warm the olive oil in a skillet over medium heat. Add red onion and collard greens and cook for 7 minutes until soft.
3. Combine the remaining mustard, apple cider vinegar, salt, and pepper in a bowl. Pour in the skillet and cook for 2 minutes. Serve the pork chops with kale side.

PER SERVING

Cal 510; Fat 40g; Carbs 11g; Protein 2g

Cinnamon Pork Chops in Apple Sauce
Prep time: 5 minutes | Cook time: 45 minutes | Serves 4

- ¼ cup chopped onions
- ½ tsp grated fresh ginger
- 2 apples, peeled and diced
- 2 tbsp olive oil
- 4 boneless pork chops
- 1 tsp garlic powder
- 1 tsp ground cinnamon
- Sea salt and pepper to taste

1. Warm 1 tbsp of olive oil in a skillet over medium heat. Add the onions and ginger and sauté for 2 minutes until softened.
2. Stir in the apples. Sauté for about 5 minutes, or until the fruit is just tender. Season with salt; set it aside.
3. Sprinkle the pork chops with garlic powder, cinnamon, salt, and pepper. Warm the remaining olive oil in the skillet and add the chops. Sear them for 3-4 minutes per side until just cooked through and browned, turning once. Serve the chops drizzled with the apple sauce.

PER SERVING

Cal 430; Fat 30g; Carbs 10g; Protein 25g

Za'atar Pork Tenderloin
Prep time: 5 minutes | Cook time: 35 minutes | Serves 2

- ½ lb pork tenderloin
- 1 tsp za'atar seasoning
- Zest of 1 lemon
- 1 tsp chili powder
- ½ tsp dried thyme
- ¼ tsp garlic powder
- ¼ tsp sea salt
- 1 tbsp olive oil

1. Preheat your oven to 425°F. Place the za'atar seasoning, lemon zest, thyme, garlic powder, chili powder, and salt in a bowl and mix well. Rub the pork with the mixture.
2. Warm the olive oil in a skillet over medium heat. Add the pork tenderloin and sear for 6 minutes or until browned. Flip the pork halfway through the cooking time.
3. Place the skillet in the oven and roast for 15 minutes or until an instant-read thermometer inserted in the thickest part of the tenderloin registers at least 145°F.
4. Transfer the cooked tenderloin to a large plate and allow to cool for a few minutes before serving.

PER SERVING

Cal 185; Fat 10g; Carbs 1g; Protein 19g

Thyme Pork Loin Bake
Prep time: 5 minutes | Cook time: 90 minutes | Serves 4

- 1 lb boned pork loin
- 1 fennel bulb, sliced
- ½ celeriac, diced
- 2 tbsp olive oil
- 1 tbsp pure maple syrup
- 1 lemon, zested
- A pinch of sea salt
- 1 tsp chopped thyme

1. Preheat your oven to 375°F. Toss the fennel, celeriac, 1 tablespoon of olive oil, maple syrup, lemon zest, and sea salt in a baking dish.
2. Warm the remaining olive oil in a large skillet over medium heat and add the pork loin. Brown it on all sides, turning, for about 15 minutes total. Place the browned pork on top of the vegetables and sprinkle with thyme.
3. Roast the pork for about 1 hour until cooked through, but still juicy. Transfer the roast and vegetables to a serving platter and pour any pan juices over the top. Serve and enjoy!

PER SERVING

Cal 405; Fat 22g; Carbs 15g; Protein 32g

Pecan-Dusted Pork Tenderloin Slices
Prep time: 5 minutes | Cook time: 20 minutes | Serves 4

- 1 lb pork tenderloin, sliced
- Sea salt and pepper to taste
- ½ cup pecans
- 1 cup full-fat coconut milk
- 2 tbsp olive oil

1. Preheat your oven to 400°F. Pulse the pecans in your blender until a powder consistency is reached.
2. Remove to a bowl and mix with salt and pepper. In another bowl, combine the coconut milk and olive oil.
3. Dip the pork chops first in the coconut mixture, then in the pecan mix, and transfer to a parchment-lined baking sheet.
4. Bake for 10 minutes until the meat reaches an internal temperature of 160°F. Serve immediately.

PER SERVING

Cal 440; Fat 35g; Carbs 7g; Protein 4g

Rosemary Pork Loin

Prep time: 15 minutes | Cook time: 60 minutes | Serves 4

- 2 tbsp olive oil
- 2 lb boneless pork loin
- 1 tsp dried rosemary
- Sea salt and pepper to taste

1. Preheat your oven to 375°F. Pour 1 cup of water into a roasting pan. Rub the pork loin with olive oil and place it in a skillet over medium heat.
2. Cook for 4-6 minutes on all sides until browned. Transfer to the roasting pan, sprinkle with rosemary, salt, and pepper, and bake for 40 minutes. Let sit and serve.

PER SERVING

Cal 492; Fat 20g; Carbs 0g; Protein 76g

Worcestershire Pork Chops

Prep time: 5 minutes | Cook time: 35 minutes| Serves 6

- 1 onion, diced
- 8 pork chops
- ¼ cup olive oil
- 3 tbsp Worcestershire sauce
- 4 sweet potatoes, diced

1. Heat half of the oil in your pressure cooker on "Sauté". Brown the pork chops on all sides and season with salt and pepper. Set aside.
2. Add the rest of the oil to the Instant Pot. Add onions and sauté for 2 or 3 minutes. Add potatoes and add 1 cup of water and Worcestershire sauce. Return the pork chops to the cooker.
3. Close the lid, press "Manual" and cook for 15 minutes. When cooking is complete, select Cancel and perform a natural pressure release. This will take about 15 minutes.

PER SERVING

Cal 785; Fat 40g; Carbs 26g; Protein 73g

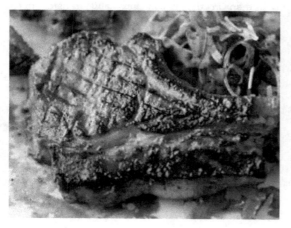

Sunday Pork Tacos

Prep time: 5 minutes | Cook time: 8 hours 15 minutes| Serves 4

- 3 lb pork shoulder
- 2 cups chicken broth
- Juice of 1 orange
- 1 small onion, chopped
- 4 coconut taco shells
- Sea salt and pepper to taste
- 1 tsp ground cumin
- 1 tsp garlic powder
- ½ tsp dried coriander

1. Rub the pork with salt, cumin, garlic powder, coriander, and pepper. Put it in your slow cooker.
2. Pour the broth and orange juice around the pork. Scatter the onion around the pork.
3. Cover the cooker and set on "Low". Cook for 8 hours. Transfer the pork to a work surface and shred it with a fork. Serve in taco shells and enjoy!

PER SERVING

Cal 1150; Fat 85g; Carbs 12g; Protein 82g

Chocolate Chili

Prep Time: 15 minutes | Cook time: 45 minutes| Serves 4

- 1 tablespoon extra-virgin olive oil
- 1 pound lean ground beef
- 1 large onion, chopped
- 2 garlic cloves, minced
- 1 tablespoon unsweetened cocoa
- 1½ teaspoons chili powder
- 1 teaspoon salt
- ½ teaspoon ground cumin
- 2 cups chicken broth
- 1 cup tomato sauce

1. In a Dutch oven, heat the oil over high heat. Add the ground beef and brown well, about 5 minutes.
2. Add the onion, garlic, cocoa, chili powder, salt, and cumin and cook, stirring, for an additional minute.
3. Add the chicken broth and tomato sauce and bring to a boil. Reduce the heat to a simmer, cover, and cook, stirring occasionally, for 30 to 40 minutes. If the sauce becomes too thick as it cooks, add more chicken broth or water to thin it.
4. Ladle into bowls and serve.

PER SERVING

Calories: 370; Total Fat: 27g; Total Carbohydrates: 9g; Sugar: 4g; Fiber: 2g; Protein: 23g; Sodium: 1,010mg

Spicy Lime Pork Tenderloins

Prep time: 5 minutes | Cook time: 7 hours 15 minutes| Serves 4

- 2 lb pork tenderloins
- 1 cup chicken broth
- ¼ cup lime juice
- 3 tsp chili powder
- 2 tsp garlic powder
- 1 tsp ginger powder
- ½ tsp sea salt

1. Combine chili powder, garlic powder, ginger powder, and salt in a bowl.
2. Rub the pork all over with the spice mixture and put it in your slow cooker. Pour in the broth and lime juice around the pork.
3. Cover with the lid and cook for 7 hours on "Low". Remove the pork from the slow cooker and let rest for 5 minutes. Slice the pork against the grain into medallions before serving.

PER SERVING

Cal 260; Fat 6g; Carbs 5g; Protein 49g

Chili Pork Ragout

Prep time: 5 minutes | Cook time: 8 hours and 15 minutes| Serves 4

- 1 cup spinach, minced
- 1 lb pork tenderloin
- 1 yellow onion, diced
- 1 red bell pepper, diced
- 1 can diced tomatoes
- 2 tsp chili powder
- 1 tsp garlic powder
- ½ tsp ground cumin
- 1 tsp fennel seeds
- ¼ tsp red pepper flakes

1. Add the pork, onion, bell pepper, tomatoes, chili powder, garlic powder, cumin, fennel seeds, red pepper flakes, and spinach in your slow cooker.
2. Cover the cooker and set to "Low". Cook for 7-8 hours. Transfer the pork loin to a cutting board and shred with a fork.
3. Return it to the slow cooker, stir it into the sauce, and serve.

PER SERVING

Cal 290; Fat 10g; Carbs 15g; Protein 35g

Garlic-Mustard Steak

Prep Time: 10 Minutes, Plus 30 Minutes To Marinate | Cook Time: 10 minutes| Serves 4

- ½ cup extra-virgin olive oil
- ½ cup balsamic vinegar
- 2 tablespoons Dijon mustard
- 2 garlic cloves, minced
- 1 teaspoon chopped fresh rosemary
- 1 teaspoon salt
- ¼ teaspoon freshly ground black pepper
- 4 (6-ounce) boneless grass-fed steaks, about ½ inch thick

1. In a shallow baking dish, whisk together the olive oil, balsamic vinegar, Dijon, garlic, rosemary, salt, and pepper.
2. Add the steaks and turn them to coat well with the marinade. Cover and let the steaks marinate for 30 minutes at room temperature or up to 2 hours in the refrigerator.
3. Heat a large skillet over high heat.
4. Remove the steaks from the marinade and blot them with a paper towel to remove any excess marinade.
5. Cook the steaks, flipping once, until nicely browned, 2 to 3 minutes on each side.
6. Let the steaks rest for 5 minutes before serving.

PER SERVING

Calories: 480; Total Fat: 31g; Total Carbohydrates: 3g; Sugar: 2g; Fiber: 0g; Protein: 48g; Sodium: 390mg

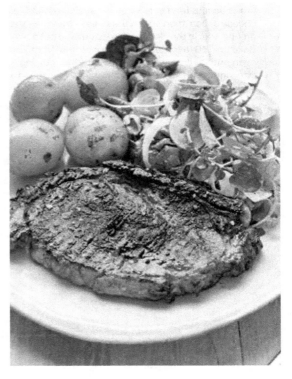

Savory Meat Pie

Prep time: 5 minutes | Cook time:45 minutes| Makes one 8-inch pie (8 servings)

- 1 pie crust, baked in a regular or springform 8-inch pan
- 1 tablespoon avocado oil
- ½ small onion, diced
- 2 cloves garlic, minced
- 1 pound ground beef (85% lean)
- 1 teaspoon fine Himalayan salt
- 1 teaspoon ground black pepper
- ½ teaspoon ground cumin
- ½ cup cheesy yellow sauce, divided
- 2 cups rainbow slaw or any shredded vegetables

1. Preheat the oven to 350°F. Set out the prebaked pie crust. It can be freshly baked or frozen; no need to thaw.
2. Heat a large skillet over medium heat. When it's hot, add the avocado oil, onions, and garlic. Sauté until tender and aromatic, about 5 minutes.
3. Add the ground beef, salt, pepper, and cumin. Sauté until browned, breaking up the meat with a whisk or spatula. Stir in ¼ cup of the sauce and quickly use a slotted spoon to transfer the beef mixture to the pie crust. You want to leave behind the pooling liquid in the skillet so the crust doesn't get soggy; let each spoonful drain before transferring it to the crust. Pat the beef down so it's compact in the bottom of the pie crust.
4. Carefully drain the liquid from the skillet and then put the pan back on the burner. Place the slaw in the skillet and sauté for 5 minutes, or until lightly browned and tender. Mix in the remaining ¼ cup of cheese sauce, then spoon the cheesy slaw over the ground beef in the pie pan. Spread out and pat down.
5. Bake for 30 minutes. Remove the pie from the oven and let it cool for 5 minutes before cutting it into eight even slices (or unpanning it if you used a springform pan). Enjoy!
6. You can store slices in an airtight container or cover the entire pie in plastic wrap and store in the refrigerator for up to 6 days. Reheat in a preheated 350°F oven or toaster oven for 10 minutes, or microwave on high for 1 minute.

PER SERVING

Calories 374 ; Fat 33g ; Total Carbohydrate 3g ; Dietary Fiber 1g ; Protein 17g

Flank Steak Pinwheels

Prep time: 20 minutes | Cook time:40 minutes| Serves 4

- 1 to 1½ pounds flank steak
- ¼ cup cheesy yellow sauce
- ½ pound fresh green beans, trimmed
- ½ teaspoon fine Himalayan salt
- ½ teaspoon garlic powder
- 6 to 8 slices thick-cut bacon
- 6 sprigs fresh oregano
- 1 head garlic
- 2 tablespoons avocado oil

1. Preheat the oven to 400°F.
2. Lay the steak flat on a cutting board. Place one hand on it and press down gently. Starting at the thickest end, cut into the meat horizontally about ¼ inch from the top and slice all the way through, going under your hand. After you have a good flap cut out, you can gently pull up on the flap as you continue to cut across the steak. You will need to keep steady pressure on the knife and make sure you don't angle it too much so the thickness remains consistent. Cut until the knife comes out the other side and you have a thin, sheetlike layer of beef.
3. If your steak is not very thick, you might be able to cut it only once. If it is very thick, cut it twice so you have three thin sheets of beef.
4. Lay the slices of beef flat on the cutting board. Cover them with a piece of plastic wrap and pound them with the smooth side of a mallet or a heavy-bottomed pot to even out the thickness and to tenderize. Do not pound so hard that you make holes in the meat.
5. Smear some sauce on one slice of steak, then add fifteen to twenty green beans. Spread them out for 2 to 3 inches along the steak, starting 1 inch from the top. Sprinkle with the salt and garlic powder. Starting at the top, roll the meat inward and over the green beans. Keep rolling until you have a burritolike tube. Holding the roll closed, wrap two or three slices of bacon tightly around it. Place the roll seam side down on a large skillet or sheet pan. Repeat with the remaining steak.
6. Top each bacon-wrapped roll with a sprig of oregano. Place the rest of the oregano between the rolls on the skillet or sheet pan.
7. Trim the top off of the head of garlic so the cloves inside are exposed. Place it on top of the oregano sprigs. Drizzle the avocado oil over everything.
8. Roast for 40 minutes, or until the bacon is cooked and slightly browned.
9. Let the rolls rest for 5 minutes, then use a sharp knife to cut each roll into four slices. Serve with the roasted garlic cloves and crispy oregano, with the pan sauce spooned over them.
10. Store leftovers in an airtight container in the fridge for up to 5 days. To reheat, cover with foil and bake in a preheated 350°F oven for 10 to 15 minutes.

PER SERVING

Calories 413 ; Fat 27.2g ; Total Carbohydrate 4.3g ; Dietary Fiber 4.5g ; Protein 37.5g

Multinational Beef + Rice

Prep time: 15 minutes | Cook time:15 minutes, plus 4 hours in a slow cooker| Serves 4

- 2 tablespoons avocado oil
- 1 large onion, diced
- 3 ribs celery, diced
- 5 cremini mushrooms, sliced
- 4 cloves garlic, minced
- 2 sprigs fresh thyme
- 1½ teaspoons garam masala
- 1 teaspoon fine Himalayan salt
- 1 teaspoon ginger powder
- 1 teaspoon ground black pepper
- 1 pound stew meat
- 2 tablespoons sunflower seed butter
- 1 tablespoon red wine vinegar or coconut vinegar
- 1 cup roasted beet marinara
- 2 cups riced cauliflower
- fresh herbs or coconut yogurt, for garnish (optional)

1. Heat a large skillet over medium heat. When it's hot, pour in the avocado oil and add the onions and celery. Sauté, stirring often, until tender, about 5 minutes.
2. Add the mushrooms, garlic, and thyme sprigs. Sauté until the mushrooms are browned, 3 to 5 minutes. Add the garam masala, salt, ginger powder, pepper, and stew meat. Stir well and cook for 5 to 6 minutes, until the beef is lightly browned. Mix in the sunflower seed butter, making sure to coat the meat.
3. Transfer everything to a slow cooker. Mix in the vinegar and marinara. Cook on low for 3½ hours, then mix in the riced cauliflower and cook for 30 more minutes.
4. Serve garnished with fresh herbs or dollops of coconut yogurt. Store leftovers in an airtight container in the fridge for up to 5 days. To reheat, bring to a simmer on the stovetop.

PER SERVING

Calories 471 ; Fat 36.1g ; Total Carbohydrate 14.4g ; Dietary Fiber 5.1g ; Protein 27g

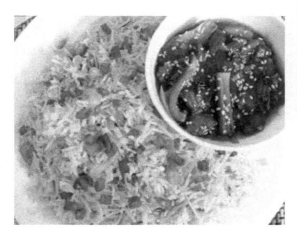

Vaca Frita

Prep time: 20 minutes | Cook time:20 minutes, plus 8 hours in a slow cooker| Serves 4

- 2 to 2½ pounds boneless chuck roast
- 2½ teaspoons fine Himalayan salt, divided
- 2 bay leaves
- 1 tablespoon white vinegar
- 3 tablespoons coconut oil or avocado oil
- 1 large onion, cut into ¼-inch slices
- Juice of 2 lemons, divided
- ½ bunch fresh cilantro, minced (½ cup), divided

1. Rub the roast with 2 teaspoons of the salt. Place in a slow cooker and add the bay leaves and vinegar. Add water until the beef is just submerged. Cook on low for 8 hours.
2. Remove the meat from the slow cooker and discard the liquid. Place the beef in a storage container, cover, and set in the refrigerator until you're ready to make and serve this dish. If you're making it right away, set the beef under a fan to cool before shredding.
3. Heat a large skillet over medium heat. When it's hot, place the oil in the skillet and add the onion slices. Cook for 10 minutes, stirring occasionally. The onions will become tender, translucent, and sweet.
4. While the onions cook, shred the meat by hand, removing any unsightly chunks of fat. Make sure to shred it into fine threads. The thinner the pieces are, the more they will crisp up!
5. Remove the onions from the skillet and set aside. Don't clean the pan. Add half of the shredded beef to the skillet over medium heat. Cook for 8 minutes, stirring once halfway through. After 8 minutes, there should be some pieces of meat stuck to the bottom of the pan; add the juice of 1 lemon and use a spatula to scrape them up.
6. Mix in half of the cilantro and half of the cooked onions. Stir to combine and immediately remove from the skillet. Repeat with the remaining shredded beef, lemon juice, cilantro, and onions.
7. Place both batches of vaca frita in a serving bowl and toss with the remaining ½ teaspoon of salt before serving.
8. Store leftovers in an airtight container in the fridge for up to 5 days. Reheat in a skillet over high heat for 5 to 10 minutes, until crispy again.

PER SERVING

Calories 639 ; Fat 50g ; Total Carbohydrate 1.4g ; Dietary Fiber 1g ; Protein 44g

Stuffed Cabbage, Dolmas-Style

Prep time: 30 minutes | Cook time:20 minutes in a pressure cooker or 1 hour on the stovetop| Makes 12 large dolmas (2 per serving)

- 1 large head green cabbage or savoy cabbage
- 2 pounds ground beef (85% lean)
- 4 cloves garlic, minced
- 1 large onion, minced
- 2 cups riced cauliflower
- ¼ cup minced fresh mint, plus more for garnish
- 1 tablespoon minced fresh oregano
- 2 teaspoons fine Himalayan salt
- 2 teaspoons ground black pepper
- 3 lemons, divided
- 1 cup water
- 2 tablespoons ghee, avocado oil, or lard

1. Turn the cabbage over so you're looking at the base. Take a paring knife and cut in an inward angle all around the core of the cabbage, then pull it out. Discard the core and set the cabbage aside.
2. Bring a large pot of water, one big enough to fit the whole head of cabbage, to a boil. While you wait for it to boil, prepare the filling: Crumble the ground beef into a large bowl. (If you don't want to handle it, you can add it to the bowl and then use a whisk to break up the beef until it's crumbled.) Add the garlic, onions, cauliflower, mint, oregano, salt, and pepper. Juice a lemon into the mix as well, catching the seeds with your hands or a fine-mesh sieve. Then use your hands to mix the ingredients thoroughly.
3. Once the water has begun to boil, squeeze the juice from a lemon into it. Use tongs to submerge the head of cabbage and hold it there for a minute or two, then let it go and cook for another 3 minutes. Use the tongs to carefully remove the cabbage from the water and set it in a bowl, cored side up. Carefully peel away the loose, tender cabbage leaves with the tongs. They should come off effortlessly; if they don't, put the cabbage back in the hot water for a few more minutes.
4. Stack the cabbage leaves on a plate or cutting board. You will need room to roll the dolmas.
5. Place a leaf in the center of your work area. Use the paring knife to trim the thickest part of the leaf, where it meets the stem, cutting out a little triangle shape. Spoon a generous amount of the meat mixture onto the leaf; the exact amount depends on the size of the cabbage, but you will get a feel for it after you've rolled one or two. With a large head of cabbage, I can fit up to a cup of filling in one dolma. Position the filling in the center toward the bottom, where you trimmed the leaf.
6. Fold the leaf upward once, then fold in the sides and continue rolling forward until you have a burrito-like roll. Make sure to apply pressure with your hands as you roll it so it stays closed. Set aside, seam side down, and repeat with the remaining filling and cabbage leaves.
7. Pressure cooker instructions:Stovetop instructions:; Use a slotted spoon to remove the dolmas from the pot. The lower ones will be delicate, so you may need to use two spoons to remove them. Serve hot, garnished with more fresh mint.
8. Unless you're feeding six adults, you will have leftovers. Store them in an airtight container, in a single layer, in the refrigerator for up to 5 days. To reheat, bake in a preheated 350°F oven for 10 to 15 minutes.

PER SERVING

Calories 361 ; Fat 22g ; Total Carbohydrate 7.6g ; Dietary Fiber 7.2g ; Protein 32g

Carne Molida

Prep time: 5 minutes | Cook time:20 minutes| Serves 4

- 2 tablespoons lard or avocado oil
- 2 pounds ground beef (85% lean)
- 1 tablespoon granulated garlic
- 2 teaspoons dried parsley
- 2 teaspoons fine Himalayan salt
- 2 teaspoons ground black pepper
- 2 teaspoons onion powder
- 1 teaspoon ground cumin
- Juice of 1 lime
- Chopped fresh cilantro, for garnish (optional)

1. Melt the lard in a large pot over medium heat. Quickly add the ground beef, crumbling it in with your hands.
2. Sprinkle all the seasonings over the ground beef and stir to combine. Use a spatula or whisk to break up the meat as you stir so that it continues to crumble and there are no large chunks.
3. Cook, stirring occasionally, for 10 to 15 minutes. The beef will brown, then release some liquid; let that liquid boil away. Increase the heat to medium-high. Keep cooking and stirring until the beef is glossy and dark brown. Once you begin having to scrape it from the bottom of the pot, it's crispy. Turn off the heat. Squeeze in the lime juice and mix.
4. Serve hot! A little chopped fresh cilantro for garnish goes really well, but it's not necessary.

PER SERVING

Calories 326 ; Fat 22.8g ; Total Carbohydrate 5.5g ; Dietary Fiber 0.7g ; Protein 24.3g

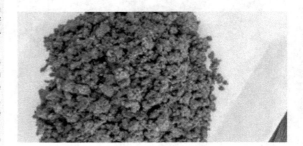

Spaghetti + Meatballs

Prep time: 20 minutes | Cook time:40 minutes| Serves 4

FOR THE MEATBALLS:

- (makes 20)
- 4 slices bacon
- 4 cloves garlic
- 3 ribs celery, roughly chopped
- 2 pounds ground beef (85% lean)
- 2 large eggs
- 2 tablespoons Italian herb blend
- 1 tablespoon fine Himalayan salt
- 2 teaspoons ground black pepper
- 2 cups roasted beet marinara
- FOR THE NOODLES:
- 2 large zucchini
- ½ teaspoon fine Himalayan salt

FOR GARNISH:

- ¼ cup shelled hemp seeds (aka hemp hearts)
- Chopped fresh parsley

1. Preheat the oven to 400°F.
2. Heat a large cast-iron skillet over medium heat. When it's hot, cook the bacon, flipping halfway through, until it has become crispy and rendered most of its fat, about 10 minutes.
3. In the meantime, place the garlic and celery in a food processor and pulse until minced. Add the ground beef, eggs, herb blend, salt, and pepper and pulse to combine.
4. Remove the bacon from the skillet, leaving the fat in the pan. Roughly chop the bacon, then add it to the food processor as well.
5. Process the bacon and beef mixture until a paste has formed. You might have to stop and use a spatula to move things along a few times. Once the meat mixture has an even texture and color, it's ready.
6. Using your hands, shape the meat mixture into 1-inch meatballs; you should get about twenty meatballs.
7. Set the skillet with the bacon fat over medium-high heat. Brown the meatballs in the bacon fat, six to eight at a time, for 6 minutes total, turning them every 2 minutes, then transfer the meatballs to a sheet pan. After all the meatballs are browned, bake them for 10 minutes to finish cooking them.
8. While the meatballs are in the oven, prepare the rest of the ingredients.
9. Heat the marinara in a large skillet over low heat.
10. Using a spiral slicer, slice the zucchini into noodles. If you do not have a spiral slicer, use a vegetable peeler to make ribbons. Toss the noodles into a bowl with the salt and set a clean kitchen towel over them, tucking the towel underneath the noodles. The towel will soak up any liquid they release. Set aside at the back of the stove or in another warm area of your kitchen to take the chill off of them.
11. In a small skillet over high heat, toast the hemp seeds for 2 to 3 minutes, moving quickly, until they begin to smell like popcorn.
12. When the meatballs are ready, remove from the oven and add twelve meatballs to the sauce, spooning a little marinara over them. Let the other meatballs cool before storing in the fridge.
13. Give the zucchini noodles a squeeze in the towel. Shake them out of the towel and divide among four serving plates. Spoon three meatballs and some sauce over each serving of zoodles and garnish with fresh parsley and toasted hemp seeds.

PER SERVING (ZOODLES WITH ½ CUP SAUCE AND 3 MEATBALLS)

Calories 425 ; Fat 29g ; Total Carbohydrate 9g ; Dietary Fiber 5.9g ; Protein 31.3g

Churrasco + Chimichurri

Prep time: 10 minutes | Cook time:16 minutes| Serves 4

- 1 pound skirt steak
- 1 teaspoon fine Himalayan salt
- 1 pound asparagus (about 15 spears)
- 1 tablespoon avocado oil
- ½ cup Chimichurri

1. Heat a large cast-iron skillet over medium heat until it's really hot, about 10 minutes.
2. Meanwhile, score the meat, making shallow cuts on the underside in a crisscross pattern. Skirt steak usually comes in foot-long strips; cut the strip into three or four pieces that fit in the skillet. Sprinkle the meat with the salt.
3. When the skillet is hot, fit as many strips of steak as you can in the skillet without overcrowding it—you may need to cook them in two batches. Sear the steak for 4 minutes on each side, or until well browned with charred bits. The meat will be crispy on the outside and medium on the inside. For medium-well steak, cook for another minute on each side.
4. When there's enough space in the skillet—usually when you're on the last batch of steak strips— throw the asparagus in there, too. Drizzle with the oil and cook for 4 minutes, turning once.
5. Serve with chimichurri spooned over everything. Store leftovers in an airtight container in the fridge for up to 4 days. To reheat, sear in a hot skillet for 2 minutes on each side.

PER SERVING (WITH 2 TABLESPOONS CHIMICHURRI)

Calories 333 ; Fat 20.8g ; Total Carbohydrate 2.3g ; Dietary Fiber 2.7g ; Protein 31.8g

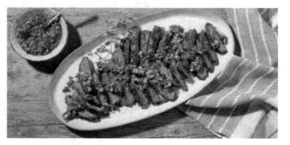

Beef Carnitas

Prep time: 20 minutes | Cook time: 20 minutes plus 10 hours in a slow cooker | Serves 8

- 4 slices bacon, diced
- 1 large onion, diced
- 4 cloves garlic, minced
- 3 to 4 pounds chuck shoulder roast
- 1 tablespoon fine Himalayan salt
- 2 teaspoons dried oregano
- 2 teaspoons ground black pepper
- 2 teaspoons ground cumin
- 3 tablespoons coconut oil
- 1 cup bone broth
- Juice of 3 limes
- ¼ cup coconut aminos
- 2 bay leaves

1. Heat a large skillet over medium-high heat. Cook the bacon, onions, and garlic in the skillet for 5 minutes, until lightly browned, then transfer the mixture to a slow cooker. Keep the skillet hot.
2. While the bacon mixture cooks, cut the roast into two equal-sized pieces and lay them flat on the cutting board. Mix the salt, oregano, pepper, and cumin in a small bowl and rub the mixture all over the roast. Scoop any seasonings left behind on the cutting board into the slow cooker.
3. Melt the coconut oil in the skillet and sear the meat for 2 minutes on all sides. Once the meat is browned, place it in the slow cooker. Pour the broth into the skillet to quickly deglaze it, scraping up any seasonings and pieces of meat that are stuck to the pan. It doesn't have to simmer, just as long as you can lift the flavorful pieces off the skillet. Pour the broth into the slow cooker.
4. Add the lime juice and coconut aminos to the slow cooker. Turn the beef over a few times in the bacon-onion mixture and broth.
5. Place the bay leaves on top of the meat and place the lid on the slow cooker. Cook on low for 10 hours.
6. Remove the meat from the slow cooker and place on a sheet pan. Use two forks to shred the beef. Pour 2 ladlefuls of liquid from the slow cooker over the beef and broil for 8 minutes, or until it reaches the desired crispiness.
7. To build the perfect taco, pile carnitas in the middle of a tortilla, spoon on some guacamole, and garnish with pickled onions.
8. Store leftovers in an airtight container in the fridge for up to 5 days or in the freezer for up to 30 days. To reheat, sauté in a skillet over medium heat.

PER SERVING (CARNITAS ALONE)

Calories 213 ; Fat 11g ; Total Carbohydrate 5.6g ; Dietary Fiber 0.8g ; Protein 23.2g

Suya Stir-Fry

Prep time: 15 minutes | Cook time: 25 minutes | Serves 4

2 tablespoons raw pumpkin seeds
2 tablespoons whole flax seeds or flaxseed meal
2 tablespoons avocado oil, lard, or unsalted butter
1 medium onion, sliced
3 cloves garlic, minced
1 pound tri-tip or sirloin steak
1½ teaspoons fine Himalayan salt, divided
1 teaspoon garlic powder
1 teaspoon ginger powder
1 teaspoon ground black pepper
¼ teaspoon ground cloves
½ cup bone broth
2 tablespoons coconut aminos
½ teaspoon liquid smoke (optional)
½ pound fresh green beans, trimmed and halved

1. Place the seeds in a coffee grinder, blender, or mortar and pestle and grind to a coarse crumble. Set aside.
2. Heat a large skillet over medium heat. When it's hot, add the avocado oil, onions, and garlic. Sauté, stirring occasionally, until tender, about 8 minutes.
3. Meanwhile, cut the beef into ½-inch pieces and place in a bowl with ¾ teaspoon of the salt, the garlic power, ginger powder, pepper, ground cloves, and ground seeds. Toss to combine and coat the beef.
4. When the onion is tender, add the beef and all of the seedy seasoning mix to the skillet. Sauté, stirring often, until the meat is browned, about 8 minutes. As you stir, a lot of the seasoning will begin to stick to the bottom of the skillet; that's okay.
5. Stir in the broth, coconut aminos, and liquid smoke (if using) and bring to a quick simmer. Use a spoon or spatula to gently scrape all the seasonings off of the bottom of the skillet and stir them in.
6. Add the green beans to the skillet and sauté, stirring often, for another 4 to 5 minutes. Sprinkle in the remaining ¾ teaspoon of salt.
7. Stir well and serve! Store leftovers in an airtight container in the fridge for up to 5 days. Reheat in a skillet over medium heat for 5 minutes or in the microwave on high for 1 to 2 minutes.

PER SERVING

Calories 410 ; Fat 26.9g ; Total Carbohydrate 15.4g ; Dietary Fiber 6.1g ; Protein 28.2g

Bacon-Wrapped Meatloaf

Prep time: 10 minutes | Cook time:50 minutes| Serves 6

- 1½ pounds ground beef (85% lean)
- ½ large red onion, minced
- 4 cloves garlic, minced
- 2 teaspoons dry mustard
- 2 teaspoons garlic powder
- 1½ teaspoons fine Himalayan salt
- 1 teaspoon ground black pepper
- 1 teaspoon onion powder
- 2 tablespoons avocado oil
- 2 tablespoons flaxseed meal
- 2 tablespoons red wine vinegar
- ½ pound bacon (7 or 8 slices)

1. Preheat the oven to 400°F. Line a sheet pan with parchment paper.
2. Place the ground beef, onions, garlic, dry mustard, garlic powder, salt, pepper, and onion powder in a large bowl and mix thoroughly to combine.
3. Add the avocado oil, flaxseed meal, and vinegar and mix again until thoroughly combined.
4. On one side of the sheet pan, shape the meat mixture into a loaf about 8 inches long and 3 to 4 inches tall. Lay the bacon slices in the center of the sheet pan and line them up so the sides overlap by ¼ inch. Lay the meatloaf in the center of the bacon. Bring the bacon slices up, wrapping them around the meatloaf and creating a seam at the top. Make sure to wrap tightly. Quickly flip the meatloaf over so the bacon seam is on the bottom. Fix the bacon slices if needed to make sure there are no gaps.
5. Bake the meatloaf for 50 minutes, or until the bacon is browned and crispy. Remove from the oven and let cool for 10 minutes.
6. Cut the meatloaf into slices the same width as the bacon slices. Serve right away.
7. Store leftovers in an airtight container in the fridge for up to a week. Reheat the slices in a skillet over medium heat until warm.

PER SERVING (1.5 SLICES)

Calories 523 ; Fat 39.2g ; Total Carbohydrate 4.9g ; Dietary Fiber 1.8g ; Protein 36.6g

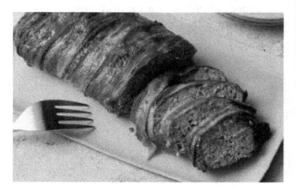

Braised Short Ribs

Prep time: 15 minutes, plus at least 30 minutes to marinate | Cook time:3½ hours| Serves 6

- 3 to 4 pounds English-cut short ribs
- ½ cup Greek Marinade + Dressing
- ½ cup diced celery
- ½ cup diced red onions
- 4 cloves garlic, minced
- 3 teaspoons fine Himalayan salt, divided
- 2 teaspoons dried rosemary needles
- 2 teaspoons ground black pepper, divided
- 3 cups shredded cabbage or collard greens
- 1 cup frozen blueberries
- 2 cups bone broth
- ¼ cup red wine vinegar
- 2 tablespoons nutritional yeast, for garnish (optional)
- Special equipment:
- Dutch oven

1. In a large bowl, toss the short ribs with the marinade. Cover and put in the refrigerator to marinate for at least 30 minutes or up to overnight.
2. Preheat the oven to 325°F.
3. Heat a Dutch oven over medium heat. When it's hot, use tongs to remove the short ribs from the marinade and place them in the pot, reserving the marinade. Brown the short ribs on all sides, about 3 minutes per side. You may have to do so in batches if they don't all fit at the same time. When seared, remove from the pot and set aside.
4. The pot should have accumulated fat from the short ribs on the bottom. Add the celery and onions and sauté until translucent and aromatic. Add the garlic, 1½ teaspoons of the salt, the rosemary, and 1 teaspoon of the pepper. Cook, stirring continuously, for 2 to 3 minutes, until fragrant.
5. Add the shredded cabbage and sauté until it begins to wilt. Return the short ribs to the pot and add the reserved marinade, blueberries, remaining 1½ teaspoons of salt, and remaining teaspoon of pepper. Use the tongs to mix as well as possible. Pour in the broth and vinegar, bring to a rapid boil, and cook for 10 to 15 minutes, until the liquid has reduced by half.
6. Cover the pot and place it in the oven. Cook for 3 hours. Remove from the oven and use tongs and a spoon to shred the meat and fish out the bones. Stir well and serve! Garnish with the nutritional yeast, if desired.
7. Store leftovers in an airtight container in the fridge for up to 5 days or in the freezer for up to 30 days. To reheat, bring to a simmer on the stovetop.

PER SERVING

Calories 704 ; Fat 55g ; Total Carbohydrate 7.5g ; Dietary Fiber 1.9g ; Protein 47g

Saucy Seasoned Liver

Prep time: 10 minutes | Cook time:8 minutes| Serves 4

- 1 pound pastured beef liver, cut into ½-inch cubes
- 1 sweet onion, thinly sliced
- Juice of 2 limes
- 1 teaspoon granulated garlic
- 1 teaspoon ground black pepper
- 2 tablespoons ghee or other cooking fat
- 1 tablespoon coconut aminos
- 1 tablespoon Dijon mustard
- 1 teaspoon fine Himalayan salt
- 1 recipe tender kale salad, for serving

1. Heat a large skillet over medium heat.
2. While the skillet heats up, place the liver, onion slices, lime juice, granulated garlic, and pepper in a large bowl. Toss to combine and let the liver marinate for a few minutes.
3. When the skillet is hot, melt the ghee. Remove the liver from the marinade, reserving the onions and marinade, and place the liver in the skillet. Sauté, stirring occasionally, for about 5 minutes.
4. Add the onions and marinade and continue to sauté for another 3 minutes. Liver should be cooked to medium, brown on the outside and just pink in the center. Well-done liver is very tough to chew.
5. Stir in the coconut aminos and mustard. Remove from the heat, sprinkle with the salt, and serve right away with the salad.
6. I do not recommend storing liver; reheating would overcook it, making it tough and chewy.

PER SERVING (WITHOUT SALAD)

Calories 227 ; Fat 10.6g ; Total Carbohydrate 8.4g ; Dietary Fiber 0.9g ; Protein 23.7g

Party Meatballs

Prep time: 20 minutes | Cook time:10 minutes| Makes 50 mini meatballs (5 per serving)

- 2 pounds ground beef (85% lean)
- 3 large egg whites, beaten
- 2 tablespoons red wine vinegar
- 1 tablespoon nutritional yeast
- 2 teaspoons dried dill weed
- 2 teaspoons dried parsley
- 2 teaspoons fine Himalayan salt
- 2 teaspoons garlic powder
- 2 teaspoons ground black pepper
- 2 teaspoons onion powder
- 1 cup coconut oil or other cooking fat, or more if needed, for frying
- Ranch Dressing or Fiesta Guacamole, for serving (optional)

1. Arrange the oven racks in the middle and bottom positions. Preheat the oven to 400°F. Line two sheet pans with parchment paper.
2. Place all the ingredients except the coconut oil and

dressing in a large bowl. Mix well with your hands. Shape the meat mixture into ½-inch meatballs. Use a small scoop or teaspoon to measure, then roll them between your hands to shape them. Place on the prepared sheet pans and bake for 10 minutes.
3. While the meatballs bake, heat a large pot over medium-high heat. Pour in the coconut oil—it should be 1 inch deep—and heat until the oil sizzles around the end of a wooden spoon handle when it's inserted in the oil. Add about fifteen meatballs at a time to the pot and cook for 3 to 5 minutes, using a slotted spoon to move and turn the meatballs as they cook. Then use the spoon to remove them from the oil and set on a paper towel–lined plate to drain. Repeat until all of the meatballs are browned and crispy.
4. Serve the meatballs with toothpicks and ranch dressing, guacamole, or another sauce for dipping, if desired.
5. Store leftovers in an airtight container in the fridge for up to 5 days. To reheat, bake in a preheated 350°F oven for 10 minutes.

PER SERVING

Calories 305 ; Fat 24.5g ; Total Carbohydrate 0.8g ; Dietary Fiber 0.6g ; Protein 20.2g

Sticky Pistou Meatballs

Prep time: 10 minutes | Cook time:25 minutes| Makes 12 meatballs (2 per serving)

- 1⅓ pounds ground beef (85% lean)
- ¼ cup Pistou
- 2 tablespoons unflavored grass-fed beef gelatin
- 1 teaspoon ground cumin
- ½ teaspoon fine Himalayan salt

1. Preheat the oven to 425°F. Line a sheet pan with parchment paper.
2. Crumble the ground beef into a large bowl. Add the remaining ingredients and mix with your hands until well combined.
3. Shape the meat mixture into twelve 2-inch meatballs and place them on the prepared sheet pan. Bake for 15 minutes, use tongs to gently turn the meatballs over, and then bake for another 10 minutes. Remove from the oven and serve hot.
4. Store leftover meatballs in an airtight container in the refrigerator for up to 5 days. To reheat, microwave on high for 1 minute or sauté over medium heat for 8 minutes.

PER SERVING

Calories 470 ; Fat 34.5g ; Total Carbohydrate 0.1g ; Dietary Fiber 0.6g ; Protein 38g

Gyro Skillet Sausages

Prep time: 20 minutes | Cook time:45 minutes| Makes 12 sausages (2 per serving)

- 1 pound ground beef (85% lean)
- 1 pound ground lamb
- 1 tablespoon dried oregano
- 2 teaspoons fine Himalayan salt
- 2 teaspoons ground black pepper
- 1 teaspoon ground cumin
- 1 small onion, roughly chopped
- ½ cup chopped fresh parsley or cilantro
- 2 large eggs
- 2 tablespoons coconut flour
- 1 tablespoon cooking fat, or more if needed

1. In a large bowl, mix together the ground beef and lamb using your hands. Add the oregano, salt, pepper, and cumin and mix thoroughly. Set aside.
2. Place the onions, parsley, and eggs in a food processor or blender. Pulse until the parsley and onion are finely minced and almost pureed. Add this to the meat mixture along with the coconut flour. Mix thoroughly.
3. Heat a large cast-iron skillet over medium heat. While it heats, shape the sausages: Take about ¼ cup of the meat mixture and roll it into a cylindrical shape no more than 2 inches in diameter and 3 inches long. Repeat with the rest of the meat mixture.
4. When the sausages are ready and the skillet is hot, heat the cooking fat in the skillet. Add four sausages, or as many as will fit without crowding the pan, and cook for 15 minutes, using tongs to gently turn the sausages every 3 to 5 minutes so they brown on all sides. When they have a nice dark crust on all sides, transfer them to a paper towel–lined plate.
5. Repeat with the next two batches of sausages, adding more cooking fat as needed between batches. There might be quite a bit of splatter, so use a splatter screen if you have one to avoid a mess.
6. Store leftovers in an airtight container in the fridge for up to 4 days. To reheat, bake in a preheated 350°F oven for 5 minutes.

PER SERVING

Calories 312 ; Fat 18.4g ; Total Carbohydrate 2.2g ; Dietary Fiber 2.3g ; Protein 32.7g

Protein Fried Rice

Prep time: 10 minutes | Cook time:25 minutes| Serves 6

- 1 pound ground beef (85% lean)
- 1 pound ground pork
- 3 tablespoons sesame oil, divided
- 3 tablespoons coconut aminos, divided
- 1 tablespoon coconut oil or lard
- 3 ribs celery, diced
- 3 cloves garlic, minced
- 2 green onions, sliced
- 1 tablespoon peeled and minced fresh ginger
- ½ cup chopped asparagus spears
- 1 tablespoon fish sauce
- 1 teaspoon fine Himalayan salt
- 1 teaspoon ground black pepper
- 1 teaspoon onion powder
- 1½ cups riced cauliflower
- Sesame seeds, for garnish (optional)

1. In a large bowl, mix together the ground beef and pork using your hands. Pour in 1 tablespoon of the sesame oil and 1 tablespoon of the coconut aminos. Gently mix and set aside.
2. Heat a large skillet over medium heat. When it's hot, melt the coconut oil in the skillet. Add the celery, garlic, green onions, and ginger. Sauté, stirring often, for 5 minutes, then remove the mixture from the skillet and set aside. Don't wash the skillet.
3. Add the meat mixture to the skillet, using your fingers to crumble it. Cook, using a whisk to break it up and stir it frequently, until browned and crumbled, 3 to 5 minutes. Continue to cook, stirring occasionally, until any fluid the meat released has evaporated, about another 10 minutes. It will smell divine, and there will be dark brown bits among the meat.
4. Add the cooked aromatics to the skillet, along with the asparagus, the remaining 2 tablespoons of sesame oil, the remaining 2 tablespoons of coconut aminos, the fish sauce, salt, pepper, and onion powder. Immediately mix in the riced cauliflower, stir, and cook for another 5 minutes, until the rice is thoroughly combined and heated. Garnish with sesame seeds, if desired.
5. Serve hot! Store leftovers in an airtight container in the fridge for up to 5 days. To reheat, sauté in a skillet over medium heat.

PER SERVING

Calories 463 ; Fat 35.3g ; Total Carbohydrate 6.6g ; Dietary Fiber 3g ; Protein 30.2g

Pan-Seared Rib-Eye with Arugula

Prep time: 5 minutes | Cook time:15 minutes| Serves 4

- 1 (1½- to 2-pound) bone-in rib-eye steak
- 2 tablespoons ghee or lard, divided
- 2 teaspoons fine Himalayan salt
- 5 cloves garlic, peeled
- 3 sprigs fresh oregano, thyme, or sage
- 2 cups fresh arugula

1. Set the rib-eye out to come to room temperature about 30 minutes before you begin cooking.
2. Place a large cast-iron skillet in the oven and preheat the oven to 425°F.
3. While the oven heats, brush the steak with 1 tablespoon of the ghee and sprinkle it with the salt.
4. When the oven has come to temperature, remove the skillet and set it on the stovetop over medium heat. Place the steak in the skillet and sear for 2 minutes. Flip the steak with tongs and top it with the garlic and herbs. Sear for 2 minutes on the other side, then place the skillet with the steak in the oven for 8 to 10 minutes, depending on the thickness of the steak and the desired doneness.
5. Remove the skillet from the oven and return it to the stovetop over medium heat. Move the herbs and garlic to the side of the pan and dollop the remaining tablespoon of ghee over them.
6. Carefully tilt the skillet so the fat pools with the garlic and herbs. Using a small spoon, repeatedly pour this pooled fat over the steak as it cooks for 2 minutes.
7. Remove the steak from the skillet and set it on a cutting board to rest for 5 minutes. When ready to serve, run a sharp knife along the inside of the bone to separate the meat, then slice the steak against the grain in very thin slices.
8. Divide the steak slices among four plates. Add ½ cup arugula to each plate and spoon the pan sauce all over the arugula. Enjoy!
9. It's a shame to eat meat this good as leftovers—it's just not the same. But if you have extra, cut it up into small pieces and store in an airtight container in the fridge for up to 4 days. Reheat in a hot skillet. Rib-eye is fatty, so it will be nice and crispy; toss it with eggs or greens for a beef hash.

PER SERVING

Calories 586 ; Fat 47g ; Total Carbohydrate 2g ; Dietary Fiber 0g ; Protein 38g

Lazy Moco

Prep time: 10 minutes | Cook time:15 minutes| Serves 4

- 4 cups riced cauliflower
- 2 tablespoons bacon fat, lard, or ghee, divided
- 2 teaspoons fine Himalayan salt, divided
- 1 pound ground beef (85% lean)
- FOR THE GRAVY:
- 3 tablespoons ghee or lard
- 2 tablespoons coconut flour
- 1 cup bone broth
- 1 tablespoon coconut vinegar
- 3 sprigs fresh thyme or rosemary
- ½ teaspoon fine Himalayan salt
- ½ teaspoon ground black pepper
- 4 large eggs

1. Preheat the oven to 425°F.
2. Spread the cauliflower on a sheet pan so that it takes up about three-quarters of it. Drizzle 1 tablespoon of the bacon fat over the cauliflower and sprinkle with 1 teaspoon of the salt.
3. Form the beef into four patties about ¼ inch thick and make an indentation in the center of each patty. Coat the patties with the remaining tablespoon of fat and sprinkle with the remaining teaspoon of salt. Line them up next to the riced cauliflower in the empty space on the sheet pan. Place in the oven and roast for 15 minutes.
4. Meanwhile, make the gravy: Melt the ghee in a small saucepan over medium-high heat. Whisk in the coconut flour and keep whisking until the flour is browned and smells toasty, almost like popcorn. This will take only a few minutes. Then pour in the broth and vinegar and stir until the mixture is smooth and fluid. Add the thyme sprigs, salt, and pepper and bring to a boil. Reduce the gravy for 5 to 8 minutes, whisking occasionally, until it becomes thick. When it's ready, it will coat a back of a spoon. Remove the gravy from the heat and discard the thyme sprigs.
5. When the patties have about 5 minutes left to cook, heat a large skillet over medium heat. When it's hot, lightly grease the skillet, then crack in the eggs. Cook, undisturbed, until the whites are cooked through. Remove from the heat. Use the edge of the spatula to separate the eggs.
6. Assemble four plates, each with a cup of riced cauliflower topped with a burger patty, a generous amount of gravy over the patty, and a fried egg. Enjoy!
7. Store leftovers in an airtight container in the fridge for up to 5 days. To reheat, place in a skillet over medium heat, and fry the egg to order.

PER SERVING

Calories 541 ; Fat 45.2g ; Total Carbohydrate 8.5g ; Dietary Fiber 5.1g ; Protein 30.9g

Slow Cooker Shawarma

Prep time: 10 minutes, plus overnight to marinate | Cook time: 8 hours in a slow cooker | Serves 6

- 1 tablespoon fine Himalayan salt
- 1 tablespoon ground black pepper
- 1 tablespoon ground cumin
- 1 teaspoon ground cardamom
- ½ teaspoon ground nutmeg
- 3 pounds boneless chuck short rib or shoulder
- ¼ cup coconut vinegar or red wine vinegar
- 3 tablespoons avocado oil
- 5 cloves garlic, peeled
- 1 large onion, quartered
- 1 lemon, quartered
- 1 navel orange, quartered

1. In a small bowl, mix together the salt, pepper, cumin, cardamom, and nutmeg. Rub the spice mixture all over the meat.
2. Place the meat in a large bowl and drizzle the vinegar and oil all over it. Add the garlic, onion, and citrus. Toss to combine, squeezing some juice out of the fruit. Cover and set in the refrigerator to marinate overnight.
3. When you're ready to cook, put everything in the slow cooker, meat on the bottom, citrus and onion quarters on top. Cook on low for 8 hours.
4. Discard the large pieces of citrus. Use two forks to shred the beef. If you like crispy beef, you can spread it on a sheet pan and broil it for 5 minutes to get delicious crispy tips. Divide the shredded beef among five or six plates, spoon the delicious slow cooker sauce over the meat, and serve.
5. Store leftovers in an airtight container in the fridge for up to 5 days or in the freezer for up to 30 days. To thaw and reheat, place in a preheated 400°F oven for 10 to 20 minutes.

PER SERVING (5 SERVINGS)

Calories 496 ; Fat 28.1g ; Total Carbohydrate 7.9g ; Dietary Fiber 1.6g ; Protein 53.9g

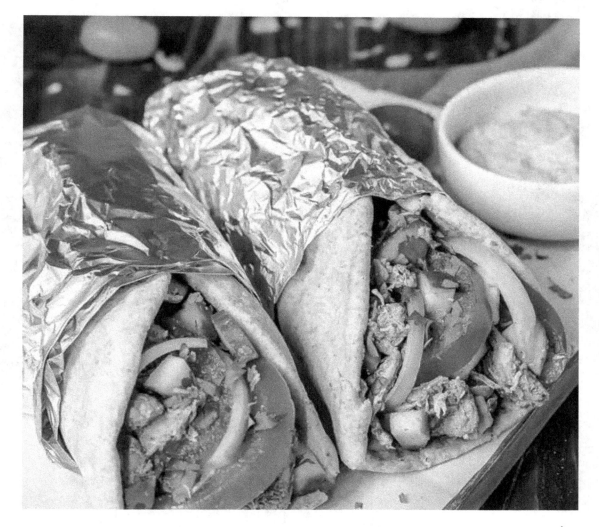

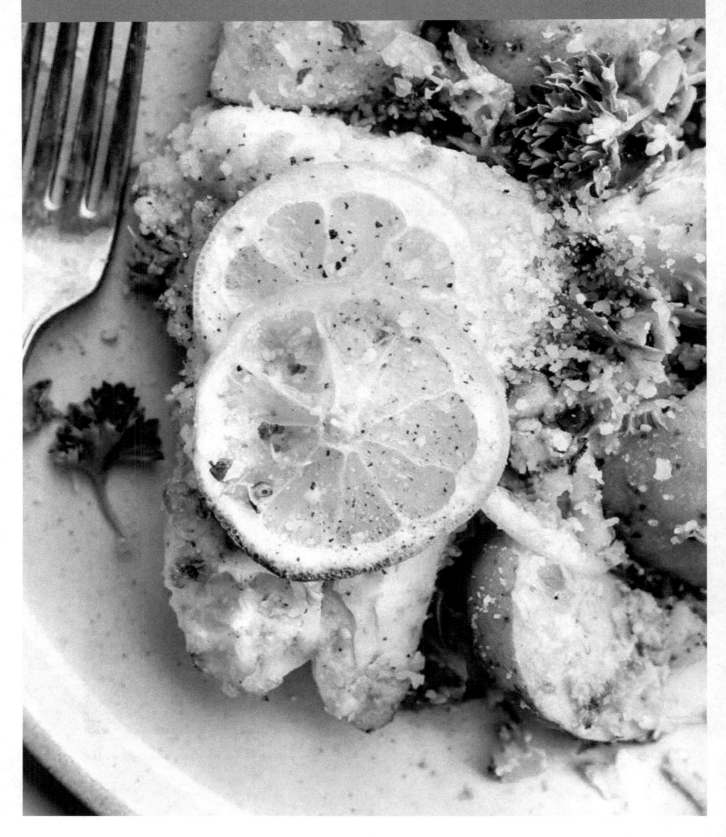

Chapter 9
Seafood Dishes

Chipotle Trout with Spinach

Prep time: 5 minutes | Cook time: 25 Minutes | Serves 4

- 2 tbsp olive oil
- 10 oz spinach
- ½ red onion, sliced
- 4 trout fillets, boneless
- 2 tbsp lemon juice
- ¼ tsp garlic powder
- ¼ tsp chipotle powder
- 1 tsp sea salt

1. Preheat your oven to 375°F. Grease a baking pan with olive oil and place the spinach and red onion on the bottom.
2. Add in trout fillets, chipotle powder, garlic, and salt and bake covered with foil for 15 minutes. Sprinkle with lemon juice and serve.

PER SERVING

Cal 162; Fat 8g; Carbs 6g; Protein 19g

Lobster & Parmesan Pasta

Prep time: 5 minutes | Cook time: 25 minutes | Serves 4

- 1 tbsp whole-wheat flour
- 8 oz whole-wheat ziti
- 1 cup plain yogurt
- 1 tbsp chopped tarragon
- ¾ cup Parmesan cheese
- 3 lobster tails
- ½ cup white wine
- ½ tsp pepper
- 1 tbsp Worcestershire sauce

1. Add 6 cups of water to the Instant Pot. Add the lobster tails and ziti. Close the lid and cook for 10 minutes on "Manual".
2. Do a quick pressure release. Drain the pasta and set aside. Remove the meat from the tails, chop it, and stir into the bowl with pasta.
3. Stir in the rest of the ingredients in the Instant Pot. When the sauce thickens, add the pasta and lobster. Cook for another 1-2 minutes.

PER SERVING

Cal 440; Fat 15g; Carbs 45g; Protein 28g

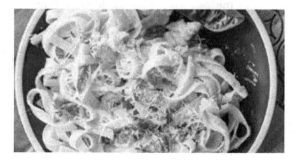

Scallops & Mussels Cauliflower Paella

Prep time: 5 minutes | Cook time: 20 minutes | Serves 4

- 1 red bell pepper, diced
- 1 tbsp coconut oil
- 1 cup scallops
- 2 cups mussels
- 1 onion, diced
- 2 cups ground cauliflower
- 2 cups fish stock
- A pinch of turmeric

1. Press the Sauté button on the Instant Pot and melt the coconut oil. Add the onion and bell pepper and cook for about 4 minutes. Stir in scallops and turmeric and cook for 2 minutes.
2. Stir in the remaining ingredients and close the lid. Cook for 6 minutes on "Manual" on high pressure. Once cooked, release a quick pressure. Serve.

PER SERVING

Cal 155; Fat 5g; Carbs 12g; Protein 7g

Shrimp & Egg Risotto

Prep time: 5 minutes | Cook time: 40 minutes | Serves 6

- 4 cups water
- 4 garlic cloves, minced
- 2 eggs, beaten
- ½ tsp grated ginger
- 3 tbsp olive oil
- ¼ tsp cayenne pepper
- 1½ cups frozen peas
- 2 cups brown rice
- ¼ cup soy sauce
- 1 cup chopped onion
- 12 oz peeled shrimp, thawed

1. Heat the olive oil in your Instant Pot on "Sauté". Add the onion and garlic and cook for 2 minutes. Stir in the remaining ingredients except for the shrimp and eggs.
2. Close the lid and cook on "Manual" for 20 minutes. Wait about 10 minutes before doing a quick release.
3. Stir in the shrimp and eggs. And let them heat for a couple of seconds with the lid off. Serve and enjoy!

PER SERVING

Cal 220; Fat 10g; Carbs 20g; Protein 13g

Creamy Crabmeat

Prep time: 5 minutes | Cook time: 15 minutes | Serves 4

- ¼ cup olive oil
- 1 small red onion, chopped
- 1 lb lump crab meat
- ½ celery stalk, chopped
- ½ cup plain yogurt
- ¼ cup chicken broth

1. Season the crabmeat with some salt and pepper. Heat the oil in your Instant Pot on "Sauté". Add celery and onion and cook for 3 minutes, or until soft.
2. Add the crabmeat and stir in the broth. Seal and lock the lid and set to "Steam" for 5 minutes on high pressure.
3. Once the cooking is complete, do a quick release and carefully open the lid. Stir in the yogurt and serve.

PER SERVING

Cal 450; Fat 10g; Carbs 12g; Protein 40g

Yummy Fish Curry

Prep time: 5 minutes | Cook time: 30 minutes | Serves 4

- 2 shallots, chopped
- 2 garlic cloves, minced
- 2 tbsp coconut oil
- 1 tbsp minced fresh ginger
- 2 tsp curry powder
- Sea salt and pepper to taste
- 2 cups cubed butternut squash
- 2 cups chopped broccoli
- 1 (13-oz) can coconut milk
- 1 cup vegetable broth
- 1 lb firm white fish fillets
- ¼ cup chopped cilantro
- 1 scallion, sliced thin
- Lemon wedges, for garnish

1. Melt the coconut oil in a large pot over medium heat. Add the shallots, garlic, ginger, curry powder, salt, and pepper. Sauté for 5 minutes. Add the butternut squash and broccoli. Sauté for 2 minutes more.
2. Stir in the coconut milk and vegetable broth and bring to a boil. Reduce the heat to simmer and add the fish. Cover the pot and simmer for 5 minutes, or until the fish is cooked through.
3. Remove and discard the lemongrass. Ladle the curry into a serving bowl. Garnish with the cilantro and scallion and serve with lemon wedges.

PER SERVING

Cal 550; Fat 39g; Carbs 22g; Protein 33g

Greek-Style Sea Bass

Prep time: 5 minutes | Cook time: 25 minutes | Serves 4

- 4 (5-oz) sea bass fillets
- 1 small onion, diced
- ½ cup vegetable broth
- 1 cup canned diced tomatoes
- ½ cup chopped black olives
- 2 tbsp capers, drained
- 2 cups packed spinach
- 2 tbsp extra-virgin olive oil
- Sea salt and pepper to taste
- 1 tsp Greek oregano

1. Preheat your oven to 375°F. Coat the fish with olive oil in a baking dish Season with Greek oregano, salt, and pepper.
2. Top the fish with the onion, broth, tomatoes, olives, capers, spinach, salt, and pepper.
3. Cover the baking dish with aluminum foil and place it in the oven. Bake for 15 minutes, or until the fish is cooked through. Serve.

PER SERVING

Cal 275; Fat 12g; Carbs 5g; Protein 34g

Fish Stew

Prep time: 5 minutes | Cook time: 30 minutes | Serves 4

- 2 lb white fish fillets, cut into 2-inch pieces
- 1 white onion, sliced thin
- 1 fennel bulb, sliced thin
- 2 garlic cloves, minced
- 1 (28-oz) can diced tomatoes
- 2 tbsp extra-virgin olive oil
- ¼ tsp turmeric
- 1 tsp ground cumin
- 1 tsp ground oregano
- Sea salt and pepper to taste
- 2 tbsp chopped parsley
- ½ lemon, juiced

1. Warm the olive oil in a large pot over medium heat. Add the onion, fennel, and garlic. Sauté for 5 minutes.
2. Stir in the crushed tomatoes, turmeric, cumin, oregano, salt, and pepper. Bring the mixture to a simmer.
3. Lay the fish fillets in a single layer over the vegetables, cover the pan, and simmer for 10 minutes. Garnish with parsley and lemon juice. Serve and enjoy!

PER SERVING

Cal 530; Fat 20g; Carbs 24g; Protein 61g

Chard Trout Fillets

Prep time: 5 minutes | Cook time: 25 minutes | Serves 4

- 2 garlic cloves, minced
- 2 bunches chard, sliced
- 4 boneless trout fillets
- Sea salt and pepper to taste
- 1 tbsp extra-virgin olive oil
- 1 onion, chopped
- 2 oz capers
- 1 tbsp apple cider vinegar
- ½ cup vegetable broth

1. Preheat your oven to 375°F. Warm the olive oil in a large pan over medium heat. Sauté the onion and garlic for 3 minutes.
2. Add the chard and cook for 2 more minutes. Add the chard, capers, cider vinegar, and broth to the pan. Season the trout fillets with salt and pepper and place them in the pan.
3. Cover and place it in the oven for about 10 minutes, or until the trout is cooked through.

PER SERVING

Cal 230; Fat 10g; Carbs 15g; Protein 23g

Hazelnut Crusted Trout Fillets

Prep time: 5 minutes | Cook time: 30 minutes | Serves 4

- 4 boneless trout fillets
- 1 cup hazelnuts, ground
- 1 tbsp coconut oil, melted
- 2 tbsp chopped thyme
- Sea salt and pepper to taste
- Lemon wedges, for garnish

1. Preheat your oven to 375°F. Place the trout fillets on a greased baking sheet skin-side down. Season with salt and pepper. Gently press ¼ cup of ground hazelnuts into the flesh of each fillet.
2. Drizzle the melted coconut oil over the nuts and then sprinkle with thyme. Bake for 15 minutes, or until the fish is cooked through. Serve.

PER SERVING

Cal 670; Fat 59g; Carbs 15g; Protein 29g

Baked Cod Fillets with Mushroom

Prep time: 5 minutes | Cook time: 30 minutes | Serves 4

- 8 oz shiitake mushrooms, sliced
- 1½ lb cod fillets
- 1 leek, sliced thin
- Sea salt and pepper to taste
- 1 lemon, zested
- 2 tbsp extra-virgin olive oil
- 1 tbsp coconut aminos
- 1 tsp sweet paprika
- ½ cup vegetable broth

1. Preheat your oven to 375°F. In a baking dish, combine the olive oil, leek, mushrooms, coconut aminos, lemon zest, paprika, and salt. Place the cod fillets over and sprinkle it with salt and pepper.
2. Pour in the vegetable broth. Bake for 15-20 minutes, or until the cod is firm but cooked through. Serve and enjoy!

PER SERVING

Cal 220; Fat 5g; Carbs 12g; Protein 32g

Gingery Swordfish Kabobs

Prep time: 5 minutes | Cook time: 35 minutes | Serves 4

- 4 thick swordfish steaks, cubed
- ¾ cup sesame seeds
- Sea salt and pepper to taste
- ½ tsp ground ginger
- 2 tbsp extra-virgin olive oil

1. Preheat your oven to 400°F. In a shallow dish, combine the sesame seeds, salt, ground ginger, and pepper. In a medium bowl, toss the swordfish with the olive oil to coat.
2. Press the oiled cubes into the sesame seed mixture. Thread the cubes onto bamboo skewers. Place the skewers on a greased baking sheet. Bake them for 10-12 minutes, turning once halfway through. Serve and enjoy!

PER SERVING

Cal 390; Fat 20g; Carbs 7g; Protein 44g

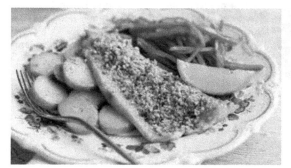

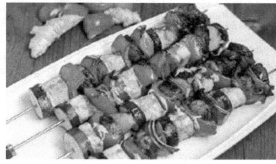

Seared Salmon with Gremolata

Prep time: 5 minutes | Cook time: 30 minutes | Serves 4

- 1 (8-oz) bag mixed greens
- 1 cucumber, sliced thin
- 1 cup watercress
- 4 salmon fillets
- 3 tsp extra-virgin olive oil
- 1 lemon, juiced and zested
- Sea salt and pepper to taste
- 1 bunch basil
- 1 garlic clove

1. Preheat your oven to 375°F. Brush the salmon fillets with some olive oil and season with salt and pepper.
2. Place in a baking dish. Add the lemon juice. Bake the fillets for about 20 minutes, or until firm and cooked through.
3. Blend the basil, garlic, and lemon zest in your food processor until everything is coarsely chopped. Arrange the greens, cucumber, and watercress on a serving platter.
4. Drizzle them with the remaining olive oil and season with salt and pepper. Place the salmon fillets on top of the greens and spread the gremolata over the salmon.

PER SERVING

Cal 275; Fat 12g; Carbs 10g; Protein 33g

Picante Trout Fillets

Prep time: 5 minutes | Cook time: 25 minutes | Serves 4

- ½ red onion, sliced
- 2 cups spinach
- 4 boneless trout fillets
- 1 tsp sea salt
- ¼ tsp chipotle powder
- ¼ tsp garlic powder
- 1 tbsp fresh mint, chopped
- 2 tbsp fresh lemon juice

1. Preheat your oven to 375°F. Spread the red onion and spinach on a greased baking pan. Lay the trout fillets over the spinach. Sprinkle the salt, chipotle powder, mint, and garlic powder over the fish.
2. Cover with aluminum foil and bake until the trout is firm, about 15 minutes. Drizzle with the lemon juice and serve.

PER SERVING

Cal 165; Fat 6g; Carbs 5g; Protein 18g

Parsnip & Tilapia Bake

Prep time: 5 minutes | Cook time: 55 minutes | Serves 4

- 2 cups diced parsnip
- 4 onion wedges
- 2 cups diced carrot
- 1 cup asparagus pieces
- 2 tsp cayenne pepper
- 1 tsp minced garlic
- ¼ tsp sea salt
- 2 tbsp olive oil
- 4 skinless tilapia fillets
- Juice of 1 lemon

1. Preheat your oven to 350°F. Take 4 pieces of aluminum foil and fold each piece in half to make four pieces.
2. In a mixing bowl, toss together the sweet potato wedges, carrot, parsnip, onion, asparagus, cayenne pepper, garlic, salt, and olive oil. Place one-fourth of the vegetables in the center of each foil piece. Top each vegetable mound with one tilapia fillet. Sprinkle the fish with lemon juice.
3. Fold the foil to create sealed packages with a bit of space at the top, and arrange the packets on a baking sheet.
4. Bake for about 30 minutes, or until the fish begins to flake and the vegetables are tender. Serve and enjoy!

PER SERVING

Cal 350; Fat 5g; Carbs 45g; Protein 35g

Olive & Salmon Quinoa

Prep time: 5 minutes | Cook time: 30 minutes | Serves 4

- 1 lb salmon fillets
- 1 red onion, diced
- 2 cups cooked quinoa
- 16 cherry tomatoes, halved
- ½ cup chopped fresh dill
- ¼ cup chopped green olives
- 1 tbsp extra-virgin olive oil
- Sea salt and pepper to taste
- 1 tbsp lemon juice

1. Preheat your oven to 375°F. Put the salmon fillets on a greased baking sheet and brush the tops with olive oil. Season with salt and pepper. Bake for 20 minutes.
2. Warm 1 tbsp of olive oil in a large pan over medium heat. Add the onion and sauté for 3 minutes.
3. Stir in the quinoa, cherry tomatoes, dill, olives, and lemon juice. Cook for 1-2 minutes, or until the tomatoes and quinoa are warmed through. Transfer the tomatoes, quinoa, and salmon to a serving platter and serve.

PER SERVING

Cal 395; Fat 15g; Carbs 36g; Protein 29g

Cumin Salmon with Daikon Relish

Prep time: 5 minutes | Cook time: 35 minutes | Serves 4

- 1 scallion, chopped
- 4 tangerines, chopped
- ½ cup chopped daikon
- 2 tbsp chopped cilantro
- 1 tsp lemon zest
- A pinch of sea salt
- 1 tsp ground cumin
- 1 tsp ground coriander
- 4 skin-on salmon fillets
- 1 tsp olive oil

1. Stir together tangerines, daikon, scallion, cilantro, salt, and lemon zest in a mixing bowl. Set the relish aside.
2. Preheat your oven to 425°F. In a small bowl, stir together the cumin and coriander. Rub the flesh side of the fillets with the spice mixture.
3. Arrange the salmon in a baking dish in a single layer, skin-side up. Brush with olive oil. Bake for 15 minutes, or until just cooked through, and lightly golden. Spoon the relish over the fish. Serve.

PER SERVING

Cal 295; Fat 11g; Carbs 14g; Protein 33g

Pan-Seared Salmon Au Pistou

Prep time: 5 minutes | Cook time: 30 minutes | Serves 3

- 2 garlic cloves
- 1 cup fresh oregano leaves
- ¼ cup almonds
- 1 lime, juiced and zested
- Zest of 1 lime
- 2 tbsp extra-virgin olive oil
- 1 tsp turmeric
- 4 salmon fillets
- Sea salt and pepper to taste

1. Spritz oregano, almonds, garlic, lime juice, lime zest, 1 tbsp of oil, salt, and pepper in your blender until finely chopped. Transfer the pistou to a bowl and set it aside.
2. Preheat your oven to 400°F. Lightly season the salmon with salt and pepper. Warm the remaining olive oil in a skillet over medium heat and add the salmon. Sear for 4 minutes per side.
3. Place the skillet in the oven and bake the fish for about 10 minutes, or until it is just cooked through. Serve the salmon topped with pistou.

PER SERVING

Cal 460; Fat 25g; Carbs 8g; Protein 48g

Persian Saucy Sole

Prep time: 5 minutes | Cook time: 40 minutes | Serves 4

- 1 red onion, chopped
- 2 tsp minced garlic
- 1 tsp grated fresh ginger
- ¼ tsp turmeric
- 2 lb sole fillets
- Sea salt to taste
- 2 tbsp lemon juice
- 1 tbsp coconut oil
- 1 cup canned coconut milk
- 2 tbsp chopped cilantro

1. Preheat your oven to 350°F. Place the fillets in a baking dish. Sprinkle it with salt and lemon juice. Roast the fish for 10 minutes. Warm the coconut oil in a pan over medium heat.
2. Add the red onion, garlic, and ginger and sauté for about 3 minutes, or until softened.
3. Stir in coconut milk and turmeric. Bring to a boil. Reduce the heat to low and simmer the sauce for 5 minutes.
4. Remove the skillet from the heat. Pour the sauce over the fish. Cover and bake for about 10 minutes, or until the fish flakes easily with a fork. Top with cilantro and serve.

PER SERVING

Cal 350; Fat 20g; Carbs 6g; Protein 29g

Gingery Sea Bass

Prep time: 5 minutes | Cook time: 15 minutes | Serves 2

- 2 spring onions, sliced
- 2 sea bass fillets
- 1 tsp black pepper
- 1 tbsp extra-virgin olive oil
- 1 tsp grated ginger
- 1 garlic clove, thinly sliced
- 1 red chili, thinly sliced
- 1 lime, zested

1. Warm the olive oil in a skillet over medium heat. Sprinkle black pepper over the fish and score the skin of the fish a few times with a sharp knife.
2. Add the sea bass fillet to the skillet with the skin side down. Cook for 5 minutes and turn over. Cook for a further 2 minutes; reserve.
3. Add the chili, garlic, and ginger to the same skillet and cook for 2 minutes or until golden.
4. Remove from the heat and add the spring onions. Scatter the vegetables and lime zest over your sea bass and serve.

PER SERVING

Cal 205; Fat 10g; Carbs 5g; Protein 24g

Fennel & Shallot Salmon Casserole

Prep time: 5 minutes | Cook time: 30 minutes | Serves 4

- 2 shallots, sliced thin
- 1 fennel bulb, sliced
- 4 salmon fillets
- Sea salt and pepper to taste
- 1 tbsp extra-virgin olive oil
- ½ cup vegetable broth
- 1 fresh rosemary sprig

1. Preheat your oven to 375°F. Brush the shallots and fennel with olive oil in a shallow roasting pan. Place the salmon fillets over the vegetables and sprinkle with salt and pepper.
2. Pour in the vegetable broth and add the rosemary sprig to the pan. Cover tightly with aluminum foil. Bake for 20 minutes, or until the salmon is cooked through. Remove and discard the rosemary sprig. Serve.

PER SERVING

Cal 290; Fat 15g; Carbs 8g; Protein 32g

Lemony Salmon with Mixed Vegetables

Prep time: 10 minutes | Cook time: 25 To 30 Minutes | Serves 4

- 4 (5-ounce) wild salmon fillets
- 1 teaspoon salt, divided
- 1 lemon, washed and sliced thin
- 1 broccoli head, roughly chopped
- 1 cauliflower head, roughly chopped
- 1 small bunch (4 to 6) carrots, cut into coins

1. Preheat the oven to 400°F.
2. Line a baking sheet with parchment paper.
3. Place the salmon on the prepared sheet.
4. Sprinkle the salmon with ½ teaspoon of salt. Drape each fillet with a few lemon slices.
5. Place the sheet in the preheated oven and bake for 15 to 20 minutes, or until the salmon is opaque and flakes easily with a fork.
6. While the salmon cooks, fill a pot with 3 inches of water and insert a steamer basket. Bring to a boil over high heat.
7. Add the broccoli, cauliflower, and carrots to the pot. Cover and cook for 8 to 10 minutes.
8. Sprinkle with the remaining ½ teaspoon of salt.
9. Top each salmon fillet with a heaping pile of vegetables, and serve.

PER SERVING

Calories: 330; Total Fat: 13g; Total Carbohydrates: 20g; Sugar: 8g; Fiber: 7g; Protein: 35g; Sodium: 761mg

Sardine Donburi

Prep time: 5 minutes | Cook time: 45 minutes | Serves 4

- 2 cups brown rice, rinsed well
- 4 cups water
- ½ teaspoon salt
- 3 (4-ounce) cans sardines packed in water, drained
- 3 scallions, sliced thin
- 1-inch piece fresh ginger, grated
- 4 tablespoons sesame oil, or extra-virgin olive oil, divided

1. In a large pot, combine the rice, water, and salt. Bring to a boil over high heat. Reduce the heat to low. Cover and cook for 45 to 50 minutes, or until tender.
2. In a medium bowl, roughly mash the sardines.
3. When the rice is done, add the sardines, scallions, and ginger to the pot. Mix thoroughly.
4. Divide the rice among four bowls. Drizzle each bowl with 1 teaspoon to 1 tablespoon of sesame oil.

PER SERVING

Calories: 604; Total Fat: 24g; Total Carbohydrates: 74g; Sugar: 0g; Fiber: 4g; Protein: 25g; Sodium: 499mg

Whitefish Chowder

Prep time: 5 minutes | Cook time: 35 minutes | Serves 6

- 4 carrots, peeled and cut into ½-inch pieces
- 3 sweet potatoes, peeled and cut into ½-inch pieces
- 3 cups full-fat coconut milk
- 2 cups water
- 1 teaspoon dried thyme
- ½ teaspoon salt
- 10½ ounces white fish, skinless and firm, such as cod or halibut, cut into chunks

1. In a large pot, combine the carrots, sweet potatoes, coconut milk, water, thyme, and salt. Bring to a boil over high heat. Reduce the heat to low. Cover and simmer for 20 minutes.
2. In a blender, purée half of the soup. Return the purée to the pot. Add the fish chunks.
3. Cook for 12 to 15 minutes more, or until the fish is tender and hot.

PER SERVING

Calories: 451; Total Fat: 29g; Total Carbohydrates: 39g; Sugar: 7g; Fiber: 8g; Protein: 14g; Sodium: 251mg

Tasty Fish Tacos with Pineapple Salsa

Prep time: 15 minutes | Cook time: 12 Minutes | Serves 6

FOR THE SALSA

- 1½ cups fresh, or canned, pineapple chunks, cut into small dice
- 1 small red onion, minced
- Juice of 1 lime
- Zest of 1 lime
- FOR THE TACOS
- 1 head romaine lettuce
- 3 tablespoons coconut oil
- 14 ounces white fish, skinless and firm, such as cod or halibut
- Juice of 1 lime
- Zest of 1 lime
- ½ teaspoon salt

TO MAKE THE SALSA

In a medium bowl, stir together the pineapple and onion. Add the lime juice and lime zest. Stir well and set aside.

TO MAKE THE TACOS

1. Separate the lettuce leaves, choosing the 6 to 12 largest and most suitable to hold the filling. Wash the leaves and pat them dry.
2. In a large pan set over medium-low heat, heat the coconut oil.
3. Brush the fish with the lime juice and lime zest. Sprinkle with the salt.
4. Place the fish in the pan. Cook for 8 minutes.
5. Flip the fish over and break it up into small pieces. Cook for 3 to 4 minutes more. The flesh should be opaque and flake easily with a fork.
6. Fill the lettuce leaves with the cooked fish (double the leaves for extra strength), and spoon the salsa over the top.

PER SERVING

Calories: 198; Total Fat: 9g; Total Carbohydrates: 12g; Sugar: 8g; Fiber: 2g; Protein: 19g; Sodium: 245mg

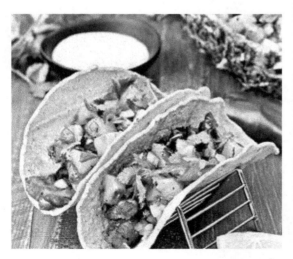

Cauliflower and Cod Stew

Prep time: 15 minutes | Cook time: 30 Minutes | Serves 4

- 3 cups water
- 1 large cauliflower head, broken into large florets (about 4 cups)
- 1 cup cashews, soaked in water for at least 4 hours
- 1 teaspoon salt
- 1 pound cod, cut into chunks
- 2 cups kale, thoroughly washed and sliced

1. In a large pot set over high heat, bring the water to a boil. Reduce the heat to medium.
2. Add the cauliflower. Cook for 12 minutes, or until tender.
3. Drain and rinse the cashews and place them in a blender.
4. Add the cooked cauliflower and its cooking water to the blender.
5. Add the salt.
6. Blend until smooth, adding more water if you prefer a thinner consistency.
7. Return the blended cauliflower-cashew mixture to the pot. Place the pot over medium heat.
8. Add the cod. Cook for about 15 minutes, or until cooked through.
9. Add the kale. Let it wilt for about 3 minutes.

PER SERVING

Calories: 385; Total Fat: 17g; Total Carbohydrates: 26g; Sugar: 7g; Fiber: 7g; Protein: 36g; Sodium: 753mg

Sautéed Sardines with Cauliflower Mash

Prep time: 10 minutes | Cook time: 15 Minutes | Serves 4

- 2 heads cauliflower, broken into large florets
- 4 tablespoons extra-virgin olive oil, divided
- ¼ teaspoon salt
- 4 (4-ounce) cans sardines packed in water, drained
- 1 cup fresh parsley, finely chopped

1. Fill a large pot with 2 inches of water and insert a steamer basket. Bring the water to a boil over high heat.
2. Add the cauliflower to the basket. Cover and steam for 8 to 10 minutes, or until the florets are tender. Transfer the cauliflower to a food processor.
3. Add 2 tablespoons of olive oil and the salt to the cauliflower. Process until the cauliflower is smooth and creamy. Depending on the size of your processor, you may need to do this in two batches.
4. In a medium bowl, roughly mash the sardines.
5. Add the remaining 2 tablespoons of olive oil to a medium pan set over low heat. When oil is shimmering, add the sardines and parsley. Cook for 3 minutes. You want the sardines to be warm, not scalding hot.
6. Serve the sardines with a generous scoop of cauliflower mash.

PER SERVING

Calories: 334; Total Fat: 24g; Total Carbohydrates: 8g; Sugar: 3g; Fiber: 4g; Protein: 26g; Sodium: 465mg

Baked Salmon Patties with Greens

Prep time: 15 minutes | Cook time: 35 To 38 Minutes | Serves 4

- 2 cups cooked, mashed sweet potatoes (about 2 large sweet potatoes)
- 2 (6-ounce) cans wild salmon, drained
- ¼ cup almond flour
- ¼ teaspoon ground turmeric
- 2 tablespoons coconut oil
- 2 kale bunches, thoroughly washed, stemmed, and cut into ribbons
- ¼ teaspoon salt

1. Preheat the oven to 350°F.
2. Line a baking sheet with parchment paper.
3. In a large bowl, stir together the mashed sweet potatoes and salmon.
4. Blend in the almond flour and turmeric.
5. Using a ⅓-cup measure, scoop the salmon mixture onto the baking sheet. Flatten slightly with the bottom of the measuring cup. Repeat with the remaining mixture.
6. Place the sheet in the preheated oven and bake for 30 minutes, flip-ping the patties halfway through.
7. In a large pan set over medium heat, heat the coconut oil.
8. Add the kale. Sauté for 5 to 8 minutes, or until the kale is bright and wilted. Sprinkle with the salt and serve with the salmon patties.

PER SERVING

Calories: 320; Total Fat: 13g; Total Carbohydrates: 32g; Sugar: 0g; Fiber: 5g; Protein: 21g; Sodium: 88mg

Sesame-Tuna with Asparagus

Prep time: 10 minutes | Cook time: 15 Minutes | Serves 4

- 2 asparagus bunches, washed and trimmed
- 3 tablespoons toasted sesame oil, divided
- ½ teaspoon salt
- 4 (4-ounce) tuna steaks
- 2 tablespoons sesame seeds

1. Preheat the oven to 375°F.
2. Line a baking sheet with parchment paper.
3. In a large bowl, combine the asparagus, 1½ tablespoons of sesame oil, and the salt. Spread the asparagus onto the prepared sheet.
4. Place the sheet in the preheated oven and bake for 15 minutes.
5. While the asparagus cooks, brush the tuna with the remaining 1½ tablespoons of sesame oil.
6. Place a sauté pan over medium heat. When the pan is hot, add the tuna. Depending on the size of your pan, you may need to cook the tuna steaks one or two at a time.
7. Sear the tuna for 3 to 4 minutes on each side, or longer if you like your tuna more well done.
8. Plate the tuna and the asparagus on four plates. Sprinkle

1½ teaspoons of sesame seeds over each serving.

PER SERVING

Calories: 349; Total Fat: 20g; Total Carbohydrates: 6g; Sugar: 2g; Fiber: 3g; Protein: 37g; Sodium: 350mg

Curry-Glazed Salmon with Quinoa

Prep time: 10 minutes | Cook time: 30 To 35 Minutes | Serves 6

- ¼ cup liquid honey
- 1 teaspoon curry powder, plus additional as needed
- 6 (4-ounce) wild salmon fillets
- 2 cups quinoa, rinsed well
- 4 cups water
- ½ teaspoon salt

1. Preheat the oven to 350°F.
2. Line a baking sheet with parchment paper.
3. In a small bowl, mix together the honey and curry powder. Taste, and add more curry powder if needed.
4. Pat the fillets dry with a clean kitchen towel and place them on the prepared sheet.
5. Brush the fillets with the curry and honey mixture.
6. In a medium pot, combine the quinoa, water, and salt. Bring to a boil over high heat. Reduce the heat to low. Cover and cook for 15 minutes.
7. Put the salmon into the preheated oven and bake for 15 to 20 minutes, or until the flesh is opaque and flakes easily with a fork.
8. Fluff the quinoa and serve alongside the salmon.

PER SERVING

Calories: 445; Total Fat: 13g; Total Carbohydrates: 48g; Sugar: 12g; Fiber: 4g; Protein: 32g; Sodium: 251mg

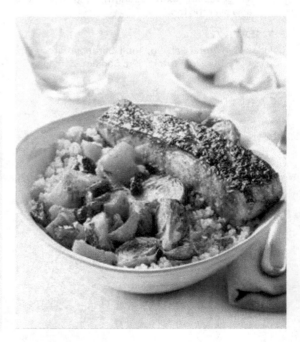

Mackerel Risotto

Prep time: 10 minutes | Cook time: 35 Minutes| Serves 4

- 8 cups Basic Chicken Broth, or vegetable broth
- 2 tablespoons coconut oil
- 1 onion, finely diced
- 4 garlic cloves, minced
- 2 cups buckwheat
- 4 (4-ounce) cans wild atlantic, King, or Spanish mackerel, drained
- ½ teaspoon salt (optional)

1. In a large pot set over medium heat, warm the broth.
2. In a second large pot set over medium heat, heat the coconut oil.
3. Add the onion and garlic. Sauté for about 5 minutes, or until soft.
4. Add the buckwheat to the pot and stir for 2 minutes to toast.
5. Add the warm broth, 1 cup at a time, stirring occasionally. When all the liquid is absorbed, add another 1 cup of broth. Repeat until the buckwheat is cooked and tender, about 25 minutes.
6. In a medium bowl, gently mash the mackerel to break it up. Fold the mackerel into the buckwheat.
7. Taste and add the salt (if using).

PER SERVING

Calories: 594; Total Fat: 31g; Total Carbohydrates: 36g; Sugar: 3g; Fiber: 5g; Protein: 43g; Sodium: 1231mg

Salmon and Mushroom Hash with Herbed Pesto

SERVES 6 Prep Time: 15 Minutes | Cook Time: 20 Minutes| Serves 6

FOR THE PESTO
- 1 bunch fresh basil
- ¼ cup extra-virgin olive oil
- Juice of 1 lemon
- Zest of 1 lemon
- ⅓ cup water
- ¼ teaspoon salt, plus additional as needed

FOR THE HASH
- 2 tablespoons extra-virgin olive oil, or coconut oil
- 6 cups mixed mushrooms (brown, white, shiitake, cremini, portobello, etc.), washed, stemmed, and sliced
- 1 pound wild salmon, cubed

TO MAKE THE PESTO
- In a food processor or blender, combine the basil (stems and all), olive oil, lemon juice, lemon zest, water, and salt. Blend until smooth.

TO MAKE THE HASH
1. In a large skillet or pot set over medium heat, heat the olive oil.
2. Add the mushrooms. Cook for 6 to 8 minutes, or until they wilt and start to exude their juices.
3. Add the salmon to the pan. Cook for 10 to 12 minutes

more, or until the salmon is cooked through.

4. Stir in the pesto. Taste, and adjust the seasoning if necessary.

PER SERVING

Calories: 265; Total Fat: 15g; Total Carbohydrates: 31g; Sugar: 7g; Fiber: 4g; Protein: 7g; Sodium: 481mg

Herbed Tuna Cakes

Serves 4 |Prep time: 15 minutes | Cook time: 30 Minutes| Serves 4

- 2 cups cooked and mashed parsnips
- 2 (6-ounce) cans wild tuna, drained
- ¼ cup almond flour, or brown rice flour
- 2 tablespoons ground flaxseed, or ground chia seed
- 1 bunch fresh parsley, stemmed and finely chopped

1. Preheat the oven to 350°F.
2. Line a baking sheet with parchment paper.
3. In a medium bowl, combine the mashed parsnips and tuna, flaking the tuna with a fork.
4. Stir in the almond flour, flaxseed, and parsley. Mix well.
5. Using a ⅓-cup measure, scoop the patty mixture onto the prepared sheet. Flatten slightly with the bottom of the measuring cup. Repeat with the remaining mixture.
6. Place the sheet in the preheated oven and bake for 30 minutes, flip-ping the patties halfway through.

PER SERVING

Calories: 273; Total Fat: 9g; Total Carbohydrates: 23g; Sugar: 4g; Fiber: 5g; Protein: 25g; Sodium: 61mg

Open-Faced Tuna-Avocado Salad Sandwiches

Serves 4 |Prep time: 10 minutes | Cook time: 0 Minutes| Serves 4

- 3 (6-ounce) cans wild tuna, drained
- 1 large avocado, halved and pitted
- 1 celery stalk, finely chopped
- ½ cup fresh parsley, minced
- 8 slices gluten-free bread, or Quinoa Flatbread

1. In a medium bowl, roughly mash the tuna.
2. Scoop the avocado flesh into the bowl with the tuna. Mash together well.
3. Stir in the celery and parsley.
4. Divide the tuna salad among 4 bread slices. Top each with a second bread slice and serve.

PER SERVING

Calories: 503; Total Fat: 25g; Total Carbohydrates: 31g; Sugar: 1g; Fiber: 7g; Protein: 35g; Sodium: 75mg

Almond-Crusted Honey-Dijon Salmon with Greens

Serves 6 | Prep time: 15 minutes | Cook time: 20 Minutes | Serves 6

- ¾ cup whole almonds
- ⅓ cup Dijon mustard, plus additional as needed
- 3 tablespoons raw honey, plus additional as needed
- 6 (4-ounce) wild salmon fillets
- 2 tablespoons coconut oil
- 3 bunches Swiss chard, washed, stemmed, and roughly chopped
- ½ teaspoon salt

1. Preheat the oven to 350°F.
2. Line a baking sheet with parchment paper.
3. Using a food processor, high-speed blender, or spice grinder, pulverize the almonds into a fine meal. If you are using a spice grinder, you may want to roughly chop the nuts first.
4. In a small bowl, stir together the mustard and honey. Taste and add more honey or mustard, if desired.
5. Put the salmon fillets on the prepared sheet. Gently pat them dry with a paper towel or clean kitchen towel.
6. Brush each fillet with the honey-Dijon mixture.
7. Sprinkle each fillet evenly with 3 tablespoons of almond meal and gently press it into the fillet with the back of a spoon or your hands. If you have any leftover almond meal, refrigerate it for another use.
8. Place the salmon in the preheated oven and bake for 15 to 20 minutes, or until the flesh is opaque and flakes easily with a fork.
9. While the salmon is cooking, heat the coconut oil in a large pan set over medium heat.
10. Add the Swiss chard. Sauté for 5 to 6 minutes, or until it is bright green and wilted. Sprinkle with the salt.
11. Remove the salmon from the oven and serve with the greens.

PER SERVING

Calories: 353; Total Fat: 21g; Total Carbohydrates: 14g; Sugar: 10g; Fiber: 3g; Protein: 28g; Sodium: 540mg

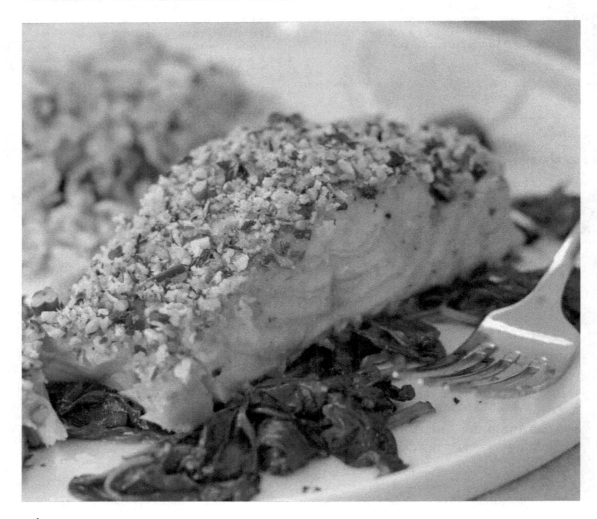

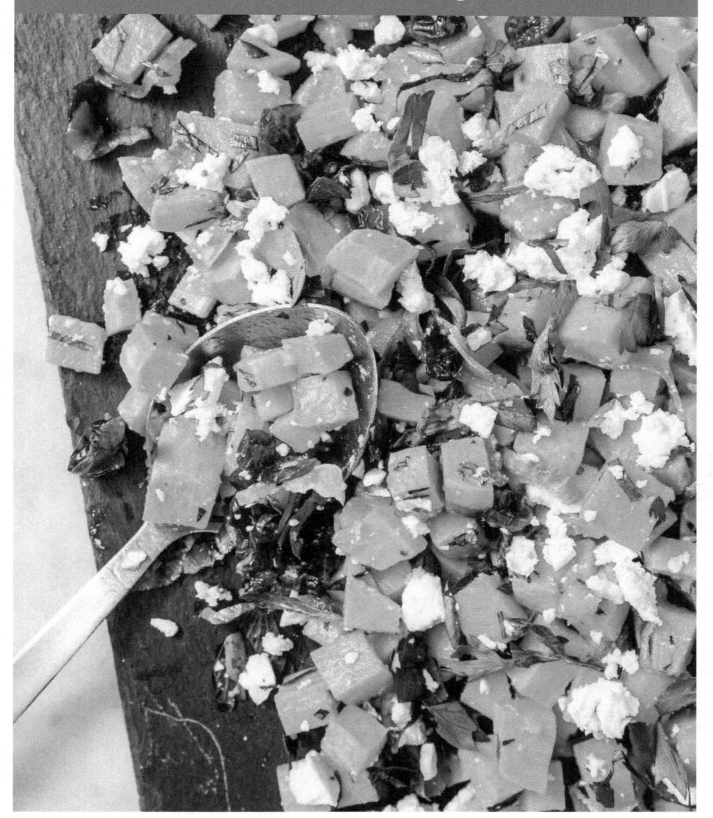

Chapter 10
Vegetarian and Vegan

Roasted Butternut Squash Soup with Sage and Pomegranate Seeds

Prep Time: 10 minutes | Cook time: 10 minutes | Serves 4

- 2 tablespoons extra-virgin olive oil
- 2 shallots, finely chopped
- 1 garlic clove, minced
- 2 cups roasted–butternut squash mash
- 2 cups vegetable or chicken broth
- ½ cup unsweetened coconut milk (optional)
- 1 teaspoon salt
- ¼ teaspoon freshly ground black pepper
- 8 fresh sage leaves
- ⅓ cup pomegranate seeds
- ¼ cup yogurt (optional)

1. In a Dutch oven, heat the oil over medium-high heat.
2. Add the shallots and garlic and sauté until softened, 3 to 5 minutes.
3. Add the butternut squash and broth and stir to combine.
4. Bring to a boil, reduce to a simmer, and cook for 3 to 5 minutes to heat through.
5. Add the coconut milk (if using) and season to taste with salt and pepper.
6. Garnish with the sage leaves, pomegranate seeds, and yogurt (if using) and serve.

PER SERVING

Calories: 200; Total Fat: 16g; Total Carbohydrates: 11g; Sugar: 4g; Fiber: 2g; Protein: 4g; Sodium: 820mg

Lentil Stew

Prep Time: 15 minutes | Cook time: 15 minutes | Serves 4

- 1 tablespoon extra-virgin olive oil
- 1 onion, chopped
- 3 carrots, peeled and sliced
- 8 Brussels sprouts, halved
- 1 large turnip, peeled, quartered, and sliced
- 1 garlic clove, sliced
- 6 cups vegetable broth
- 1 (15-ounce) can lentils, drained and rinsed
- 1 cup frozen corn
- 1 teaspoon salt
- ¼ teaspoon freshly ground black pepper
- 1 tablespoon chopped fresh parsley

1. In a Dutch oven, heat the oil over high heat.
2. Add the onion and sauté until softened, about 3 minutes.
3. Add the carrots, Brussels sprouts, turnip, and garlic and sauté for an additional 3 minutes.
4. Add the broth and bring to a boil. Reduce to a simmer and cook until the vegetables are tender, about 5 minutes.
5. Add the lentils, corn, salt, pepper, and parsley and cook for an additional minute to heat the lentils and corn. Serve hot.

PER SERVING

Calories: 240; Total Fat: 4g; Total Carbohydrates: 42g; Sugar: 11g; Fiber: 12g; Protein: 10g; Sodium: 870mg

Roasted Tri-Color Cauliflower

Prep time: 10 minutes | Cook time: 20 minutes | Serves 4

- 1½ cups white cauliflower florets
- 1½ cups purple cauliflower florets
- 1½ cups yellow cauliflower florets
- 3 tablespoons extra-virgin olive oil
- ¼ cup fresh lemon juice
- 1 teaspoon salt
- ¼ teaspoon freshly ground black pepper

1. Preheat the oven to 400°F.
2. In a large bowl, combine the cauliflower, olive oil, and lemon juice. Toss to coat well.
3. Spread the cauliflower on a rimmed baking sheet and add the salt and pepper.
4. Cover with aluminum foil and bake for 15 minutes. Remove the foil and continue to bake until the cauliflower starts to brown around the edges, about 5 minutes more.
5. Serve warm or at room temperature.

PER SERVING

Calories: 120; Total Fat: 10g; Total Carbohydrates: 7g; Sugar: 3g; Fiber: 2g; Protein: 2g; Sodium: 620mg

Quinoa With Mixed Vegetables

Prep Time: 10 minutes | Cook time: 15 minutes | Serves 4

- 3 tablespoons extra-virgin olive oil
- 1½ cups quartered Brussels sprouts
- 1 large zucchini, chopped
- 1 onion, chopped
- 3 garlic cloves, sliced
- 2½ cups cooked quinoa
- 1 cup vegetable broth or tomato sauce
- 1 tablespoon fresh lemon juice
- 1 teaspoon dried oregano
- 1 teaspoon salt
- ¼ teaspoon freshly ground black pepper

1. In a large skillet, heat the oil over high heat.
2. Add the Brussels sprouts, zucchini, onion, and garlic and sauté until the vegetables are tender, 5 to 7 minutes.
3. Add the quinoa and broth, cover, and cook for an additional 5 minutes.
4. Add the lemon juice, oregano, salt, and pepper and stir to fluff the quinoa.
5. Serve warm or at room temperature.

PER SERVING

Calories: 270; Total Fat: 13g; Total Carbohydrates: 34g; Sugar: 5g; Fiber: 8g; Protein: 8g; Sodium: 640mg

Green Pasta Salad

Prep Time: 15 minutes | Cook time: 15 minutes| Serves 4

- 1 (12-ounce) package gluten-free penne or fusilli
- 1 bunch asparagus, sliced on the diagonal into 1-inch pieces
- 1 tablespoon extra-virgin olive oil
- 1 cup tofu-basil sauce
- 2 cups arugula
- 2 scallions, sliced
- 1 teaspoon salt
- ¼ teaspoon freshly ground black pepper

1. Cook the pasta in a large pot of boiling water according to the package directions. Add the asparagus to the pot for the last 2 minutes of cooking time. Drain the pasta and asparagus in a colander, then return them to the pot.
2. Add the olive oil and sauce and stir to combine. Set aside to cool to room temperature.
3. Stir in the arugula, scallions, salt, and pepper and serve.

PER SERVING

Calories: 450; Total Fat: 15g; Total Carbohydrates: 68g; Sugar: 3g; Fiber: 5g; Protein: 13g; Sodium: 290mg

Herb Omelet

Prep Time: 10 minutes | Cook time: 5 minutes| Serves 2

- 3 large eggs
- 1 tablespoon chopped fresh chives
- 1 tablespoon chopped fresh parsley
- 1 teaspoon ground turmeric
- ¼ teaspoon ground cumin
- ½ teaspoon salt
- 2 tablespoons extra-virgin olive, divided

1. In a medium bowl, whisk together the eggs, chives, parsley, turmeric, cumin, and salt.
2. In an omelet pan, heat 1 tablespoon of oil over medium-high heat.
3. Pour half of the egg mixture into the hot pan.
4. Reduce the heat to medium and let the eggs cook until the bottom starts to set.
5. Using a heat-proof spatula, gently move the eggs around the edges so the uncooked egg can spill over the sides of the cooked egg and set.
6. Continue to cook the omelet until just set, but still soft. Use the spatula to fold the omelet in half, then slide it out of the pan and onto a serving dish.
7. Repeat with the remaining egg mixture and 1 tablespoon of oil. Serve.

PER SERVING

Calories: 240; Total Fat: 21g; Total Carbohydrates: <1g; Sugar: <1g; Fiber: 0g; Protein: 11g; Sodium: 310mg

Vegetable Curry

Prep time: 15 minutes | Cook time: 15 minutes| Serves 4

- 1 tablespoon coconut oil
- 1 onion, chopped
- 2 cups (½-inch) butternut squash cubes
- 1 large sweet potato, peeled and cut into ½-inch cubes
- 2 garlic cloves, sliced
- 1 (13.5-ounce) can coconut milk
- 2 cups vegetable broth
- 2 teaspoons curry powder
- 1 teaspoon salt
- 2 tablespoons chopped fresh cilantro

1. In a Dutch oven, heat the oil over high heat.
2. Add the onion and sauté until softened, about 3 minutes.
3. Add the butternut squash, sweet potato, and garlic and sauté for an additional 3 minutes.
4. Add the coconut milk, broth, curry powder, and salt and bring to a boil. Reduce to a simmer and cook until the vegetables are tender, about 5 minutes.
5. Top with the cilantro and serve.

PER SERVING

Calories: 120; Total Fat: 5g; Total Carbohydrates: 20g; Sugar: 4g; Fiber: 3g; Protein: 2g; Sodium: 670mg

Whole-Wheat Penne with White Beans, Chard, and Walnuts

Prep Time: 10 minutes | Cook time: 18 minutes| Serves 4

- 1 (12-ounce) package whole-wheat penne
- 2 tablespoons extra-virgin olive oil
- 1 bunch Swiss chard, cut into thin ribbons
- 1 garlic clove, sliced
- 1 teaspoon salt
- ⅛ teaspoon red pepper flakes
- 1 (15-ounce) can white beans, drained and rinsed
- ¼ cup chopped toasted walnuts (optional)

1. Cook the penne in a large pot of boiling water according to the package directions, then drain.
2. While the pasta is cooking, in a large skillet, heat the oil over high heat.
3. Add the chard, garlic, salt, and red pepper flakes and cook until the chard has wilted, about 3 minutes. Stir in the white beans until warm.
4. In a large serving bowl, toss together the penne and chard-bean mixture, mixing well. Sprinkle with the walnuts and serve.

PER SERVING

Calories: 620; Total Fat: 14g; Total Carbohydrates: 101g; Sugar: 5g; Fiber: 17g; Protein: 25g; Sodium: 660mg

Tamari Tofu with Sweet Potatoes & Broccoli
Prep time: 5 minutes | Cook time: 15 minutes| Serves 4

- 1 lb tofu, cubed
- 3 garlic cloves, minced
- 2 tbsp tamari
- 2 tbsp sesame seeds
- 2 tsp olive oil
- 2 tbsp tahini
- 1 tbsp rice vinegar
- 1 cup vegetable stock
- 1 onion, sliced
- 2 cups broccoli florets
- 1 cup diced sweet potatoes
- 2 tbsp sriracha

1. Heat the oil in your Instant Pot on "Sauté". Add the onion and sweet potatoes and cook for 2 minutes.
2. Add garlic and half of the sesame seeds, and cook for a minute more. Stir in tamari, broth, tofu, and vinegar.
3. Seal the lid and set steam vent to Sealing. Select "Manual" and cook for 3 minutes on high pressure. Release the pressure quickly, add the broccoli and seal the lid again. Cook for 2 more minutes.
4. Then, perform a quick pressure release and open the lid. Stir in sriracha and tahini before serving.

PER SERVING

Cal 250; Fat 12g; Carbs 20g; Protein 17g

Tofu Cabbage Stir-Fry
Prep time: 5 minutes | Cook time: 45 minutes| Serves 4

2 ½ cups bok choy, sliced
2 tbsp coconut oil
2 cups tofu, cubed
1 tsp garlic powder
1 tsp onion powder
1 tbsp plain vinegar
2 garlic cloves, minced
1 tsp chili flakes
1 tbsp grated ginger
3 green onions, sliced
1 tbsp olive oil
1 cup paleo mayonnaise

1. Warm the coconut oil in a wok over medium heat. Add bok choy and stir-fry until softened.
2. Season with salt, pepper, garlic powder, onion powder, and plain vinegar. Sauté for 2 minutes; set aside.
3. To the wok, add the garlic, chili flakes, and ginger and sauté them until fragrant. Put the tofu in the wok and cook until browned on all sides.
4. Add the green onions and bok choy, heat for 2 minutes, and add the olive oil. Stir in mayonnaise. Serve.

PER SERVING

Cal 200; Fat 16g; Carbs 6g; Protein 9g

Mushroom & Green Bean Biryani
Prep time: 5 minutes | Cook time: 50 minutes| Serves 4

- 1 cup chopped mushrooms
- 1 cup brown rice
- 3 tbsp olive oil
- 3 white onions, chopped
- 6 garlic cloves, minced
- 1 tsp ginger puree
- 1 tbsp turmeric powder
- ¼ tsp cinnamon powder
- 2 tsp garam masala
- ½ tsp cardamom powder
- ½ tsp cayenne powder
- ½ tsp cumin powder
- 1 tsp smoked paprika
- 3 large tomatoes, diced
- 2 green chilies, minced
- 1 tbsp tomato puree
- 1 cup chopped mustard greens
- 1 cup Greek yogurt

1. Warm the olive oil in a large pot over medium heat. Sauté the onions until softened, 3 minutes.
2. Mix in the garlic, ginger, turmeric, cardamom, garam masala, cayenne pepper, cumin, paprika, and salt. Stir-fry for 1-2 minutes. Pour in the tomatoes, green chili, tomato puree, and mushrooms. Once boiling, mix in the rice and cover it with water.
3. Cover the pot and cook until the liquid absorbs and the rice is tender, 15-20 minutes. Open the lid and fluff in the mustard greens and parsley. Top with coconut yogurt and serve.

PER SERVING

Cal 395; Fat 13g; Carbs 59g; Protein 6g

Cheesy Cauliflower Casserole
Prep time: 5 minutes | Cook time: 35 minutes| Serves 4

- 1 white onion, chopped
- ½ celery stalk, chopped
- 1 green bell pepper, chopped
- Sea salt and pepper to taste
- 1 head cauliflower, chopped
- 1 cup paleo mayonnaise
- 4 oz grated Parmesan
- 1 tsp red chili flakes

1. Preheat your oven to 400°F. Season onion, celery, and bell pepper with salt and black pepper.
2. In a bowl, mix cauliflower, mayonnaise, Parmesan cheese, and red chili flakes.
3. Pour the mixture into a greased baking dish and add the vegetables; mix to distribute. Bake for 20 minutes. Remove and serve warm.

PER SERVING

Cal 115; Fat 4g; Carbs 6g; Protein 17g

Mushroom Lettuce Wraps

Prep time: 5 minutes | Cook time: 25 minutes| Serves 4

- 4 oz baby Bella mushrooms, sliced
- 2 tbsp olive oil
- 1½ lb tofu, crumbled
- 1 lettuce, leaves extracted
- 1 cup grated Parmesan
- 1 large tomato, sliced

1. Warm the olive oil in a skillet, add mushrooms, and sauté until browned and tender, about 6 minutes.
2. Transfer to a plate. Add the tofu to the skillet and cook until brown, about 10 minutes.
3. Spoon the tofu and mushrooms into the lettuce leaves, sprinkle with the Parmesan cheese, and share the tomato slices on top. Serve immediately.

PER SERVING

Cal 530; Fat 29g; Carbs 40g; Protein 39g

White Pizza with Mixed Mushrooms

Prep time: 5 minutes | Cook time: 35 minutes| Serves 4

- 2 oz mixed mushrooms, sliced
- 2 eggs, beaten
- ½ cup paleo mayonnaise
- ¾ cup almond flour
- 1 tbsp psyllium husk powder
- 1 tsp baking powder
- 1 tbsp basil pesto
- 2 tbsp olive oil
- Sea salt and pepper to taste
- ½ cup coconut cream
- ¾ cup grated Parmesan

1. Preheat your oven to 350°F. In a bowl, add the eggs, mayonnaise, almond flour, psyllium husk powder, baking powder, and salt and whisk well. Allow sitting for 5 minutes. Pour the batter into a baking sheet and spread out with a spatula. Bake for 10 minutes.
2. In a bowl, mix mushrooms with pesto, olive oil, salt, and black pepper. Remove the crust from the oven and spread the coconut cream on top.
3. Add the mushroom mixture and Parmesan cheese. Bake the pizza further until the cheese has melted, 5-10 minutes. Serve sliced.

PER SERVING

Cal 430; Fat 30g; Carbs 27g; Protein 15g

Baked Tempeh & Brussels sprouts

Prep time: 5 minutes | Cook time: 30 minutes| Serves 4

- 3 tbsp olive oil
- 1 cup tempeh, cubed
- 1 lb halved Brussels sprouts
- 5 garlic cloves, minced
- 1¼ cups coconut cream
- 2 tbsp grated Parmesan
- Sea salt and pepper to taste

1. Preheat your oven to 400°F. Warm the olive oil in a large skillet over medium heat and fry the tempeh cubes until browned on both sides, about 6 minutes. Remove onto a plate and set aside.
2. Pour the Brussels sprouts and garlic into the skillet and sauté until fragrant. Mix in coconut cream and simmer for 4 minutes.
3. Add tempeh cubes and combine well. Pour the sauté into a baking dish and sprinkle with Parmesan cheese. Bake for 10 minutes or until golden brown on top. Serve with tomato salad.

PER SERVING

Cal 510; Fat 42g; Carbs 26g; Protein 17g

Sweet Potato & Baby Carrot Medley

Prep time: 5 minutes | Cook time: 30 minutes| Serves 4

- 1 tsp dried oregano
- 2 tbsp olive oil
- ½ cup veggie broth
- 1 onion, chopped
- 2 lb sweet potatoes, cubed
- 2 lb baby carrots, halved

1. Heat the olive oil in your pressure cooker on "Sauté" Stir in the onions and cook for 2-3 minutes until translucent.
2. Add the carrots and cook for another 3 more minutes. Add sweet potatoes, carrots, broth, and oregano.
3. Seal the lid and turn the steam vent to sealing. Select "Manual" and cook for 10 minutes on high pressure.
4. Once the cooking is complete, allow pressure to release naturally, for 10 minutes. Carefully open the lid and serve immediately.

PER SERVING

Cal 415; Fat 8g; Carbs 80g; Protein 7g

Quinoa & Veggie Burgers

Prep time: 5 minutes | Cook time: 35 minutes | Serves 4

- 4 whole-grain hamburger buns, split
- 1 cup quick-cooking quinoa
- 1 tbsp olive oil
- 1 shallot, chopped
- 2 tbsp chopped fresh celery
- 1 garlic clove, minced
- 1 (15 oz) can pinto beans
- 2 tbsp whole-wheat flour
- ¼ cup chopped fresh basil
- 2 tbsp pure maple syrup
- 4 small lettuce leaves
- ½ cup paleo mayonnaise

1. Cook the quinoa with 2 cups of water in a medium pot until the liquid absorbs, 15 minutes.
2. Heat the olive oil in a medium skillet over medium heat and sauté the shallot, celery, and garlic until softened and fragrant, 3 minutes.
3. Transfer the quinoa and shallot mixture to a bowl and add pinto beans, flour, basil, maple syrup, salt, and black pepper.
4. Mash and mold 4 patties out of the mixture. Heat a grill pan to medium heat and lightly grease with cooking spray. Cook the patties on both sides until light brown, compacted, and cooked through, 10 minutes.
5. Place the patties between the burger buns and top with the lettuce and mayonnaise. Serve and enjoy!

PER SERVING

Cal 525; Fat 18 g; Carbs 71 g; Protein 9g

Baked Tofu with Roasted Peppers

Prep time: 5 minutes | Cook time: 20 minutes | Serves 4

3 oz Greek yogurt
¾ cup paleo mayonnaise
2 oz cucumber, diced
1 large tomato, chopped
2 tsp dried parsley
4 orange bell peppers
2 ½ cups cubed tofu
1 tbsp olive oil
1 tsp dried basil

1. Preheat your oven's broiler to 450°F. In a salad bowl, combine yogurt, mayonnaise, cucumber, tomato, salt, pepper, and parsley. Refrigerate.
2. Arrange the bell peppers and tofu on a greased baking sheet, drizzle with olive oil and season with basil, salt, and pepper.
3. Bake for 10-15 minutes or until the peppers have charred lightly and the tofu browned. Serve with the prepared yogurt salad.

PER SERVING

Cal 465; Fat 32g; Carbs 18g; Protein 12g

Mushroom Pizza

Prep time: 5 minutes | Cook time: 35 minutes | Serves 4

- 1 cup chopped button mushrooms
- ½ cup sliced mixed bell peppers
- 2 tsp olive oil
- Sea salt and pepper to taste
- 1 whole-wheat pizza crust
- 1 cup tomato sauce
- 1 cup grated Parmesan
- 4 basil leaves

1. Warm the olive oil in a skillet and sauté mushrooms and bell peppers for 10 minutes until softened. Season with salt and black pepper.
2. Put the pizza crust on a pizza pan, spread the tomato sauce all over, and scatter vegetables evenly on top.
3. Sprinkle with Parmesan. Bake for 20 minutes until the cheese has melted. Garnish with basil.

PER SERVING

Cal 420; Fat 24g; Carbs 39g; Protein 30g

Zoodle Bolognese

Prep time: 5 minutes | Cook time: 45 minutes | Serves 4

- 4 tbsp olive oil
- 1 white onion, chopped
- 1 garlic clove, minced
- 3 oz carrots, chopped
- 3 cups crumbled tofu
- 2 tbsp tomato paste
- 1 ½ cups diced tomatoes
- Sea salt and pepper to taste
- 1 tbsp dried basil
- 1 tbsp Worcestershire sauce
- 2 lb zucchini, spiralized

1. Pour half of the olive oil into a saucepan and heat over medium heat. Add onion, garlic, and carrots and sauté for 3 minutes or until the onions are soft and the carrots caramelized.
2. Pour in tofu, tomato paste, tomatoes, salt, pepper, basil, and Worcestershire sauce. Stir and cook for 15 minutes. Mix in some water if the mixture is too thick and simmer further for 20 minutes.
3. Warm the remaining olive oil in a skillet and toss in the zoodles quickly, about 1 minute. Season with salt and black pepper.
4. Divide into serving plates and spoon the Bolognese on top. Serve.

PER SERVING

Cal 415; Fat 18g; Carbs 53g; Protein 15g

Roasted Butternut Squash with Chimichurri

Prep time: 5 minutes | Cook time: 15 minutes | Serves 4

- Zest and juice of 1 lemon
- ½ red bell pepper, chopped
- 1 jalapeño pepper, chopped
- 1 cup olive oil
- ½ cup chopped parsley
- 2 garlic cloves, minced
- 1 lb butternut squash
- 1 tbsp olive oil
- 3 tbsp toasted pine nuts

1. In a bowl, add lemon zest and juice, bell pepper, jalapeno, olive oil, parsley, garlic, salt, and pepper. Use an immersion blender to grind the ingredients until your desired consistency is achieved; set aside the chimichurri.
2. Slice the butternut squash into rounds and remove the seeds. Drizzle with olive oil and season with salt and black pepper.
3. Preheat a grill pan over medium heat. Cook the squash for 2 minutes on each side or until browned.
4. Remove to serving plates, scatter the pine nuts on top, and serve with the chimichurri and red cabbage salad.

PER SERVING

Cal 615; Fat 62g; Carbs 17g; Protein 2g

Sweet and Spicy Brussel Sprout Stir Fry

Prep time: 5 minutes | Cook time: 15 minutes | Serves 4

- 2 tbsp olive oil
- 4 shallots, chopped
- 1 tbsp apple cider vinegar
- Sea salt and pepper to taste
- 1 lb Brussels sprouts
- 1 tbsp hot chili sauce

1. Warm the olive oil in a saucepan over medium heat. Pour in the shallots and sauté for 2 minutes, to caramelize and slightly soften. Add the apple cider vinegar, salt, and black pepper.
2. Stir and reduce the heat to cook the shallots further with continuous stirring, about 5 minutes. Transfer to a plate after. Trim the Brussel sprouts and cut into halves. Leave the small ones as wholes.
3. Pour the Brussel sprouts into the saucepan and stir-fry until softened but al dente. Season with salt and black pepper, stir in the onions and hot chili sauce, and heat for a few seconds. Serve immediately.

PER SERVING

Cal 125; Fat 7g; Carbs 13g; Protein 5g

Basil Pesto Seitan Panini

Prep time: 5 minutes | Cook time: 15 minutes + cooling time | Serves 4

FOR THE SEITAN:
- 2/3 cup basil pesto
- ½ lemon, juiced
- 1 garlic clove, minced
- Sea salt to taste
- 1 cup chopped seitan
- FOR THE PANINI:
- 3 tbsp basil pesto
- 8 whole-wheat ciabatta slices
- Olive oil for brushing
- 8 slices tofu
- 1 red bell pepper, chopped
- ¼ cup grated Parmesan

1. In a bowl, mix pesto, lemon juice, garlic, and salt. Add the seitan and coat well with the marinade. Cover with plastic wrap and place in the refrigerator for 30 minutes.
2. Preheat a skillet over medium heat and remove the seitan from the fridge. Cook the seitan in the skillet until brown and cooked through, 2-3 minutes. Turn the heat off.
3. Preheat a panini press to medium heat. In a small bowl, mix the pesto in the inner parts of two slices of bread. On the outer parts, apply some olive oil and place a slice with (the olive oil side down) in the press.
4. Lay 2 slices of tofu on the bread, spoon some seitan on top. Sprinkle with some bell pepper and some Parmesan cheese.
5. Cover with another bread slice. Close the press and grill the bread for 1 to 2 minutes.
6. Flip the bread, and grill further for 1 minute or until the cheese melts and golden brown on both sides. Serve warm.

PER SERVING

Cal 780; Fat 43g; Carbs 80g; Protein 12g

Jalapeño Quinoa Bowl with Lima Beans

Prep time: 5 minutes | Cook time: 30 minutes| Serves 4

- 1 tbsp olive oil
- 1 lb extra firm tofu, cubed
- Sea salt and pepper to taste
- 1 yellow onion, diced
- ½ cup cauliflower florets
- 1 jalapeño pepper, minced
- 1 tbsp red chili powder
- 1 tsp cumin powder
- 1 (8 oz) can lima beans
- 1 cup quick-cooking quinoa
- 1 (14 oz) can diced tomatoes
- 2 ½ cups vegetable broth
- 1 cup grated Parmesan
- 2 tbsp chopped cilantro
- 2 limes, cut into wedges
- 1 peeled avocado, sliced

1. Heat olive oil in a pot and cook the tofu until golden brown, 5 minutes. Season with salt, pepper, and mix in onion, cauliflower, and jalapeño pepper.
2. Cook until the vegetables soften, 3 minutes. Stir in garlic, chili powder, and cumin powder; cook for 1 minute.
3. Mix in lima beans, quinoa, tomatoes, and vegetable broth. Simmer until the quinoa absorbs all the liquid, 10 minutes. Fluff quinoa.
4. Top with Parmesan, cilantro, lime wedges, and avocado.

PER SERVING

Cal 540; Fat 29g; Carbs 45g; Protein 26g

Tofu Caprese Casserole

Prep time: 5 minutes | Cook time: 25 minutes| Serves 4

- 1 cup tofu cubes
- 16 cherry tomatoes, halved
- 2 tbsp basil pesto
- 1 cup paleo mayonnaise
- 2 oz grated Parmesan
- 1 cup arugula
- 4 tbsp olive oil

1. Preheat your oven to 350°F. In a baking dish, mix the cherry tomatoes, tofu, basil pesto, mayonnaise, half of the Parmesan cheese, salt, and black pepper.
2. Level the ingredients with a spatula and sprinkle the remaining Parmesan cheese on top. Bake for 20 minutes or until the top of the casserole is golden brown.
3. Remove and allow cooling for a few minutes. Slice and dish into plates, top with some arugula and drizzle with olive oil.

PER SERVING

Cal 475; Fat 42g; Carbs 8g; Protein 8g

Tempeh Garam Masala Bake

Prep time: 5 minutes | Cook time: 30 minutes| Serves 4

- 3 tbsp olive oil
- 3 cups tempeh slices
- 2 tbsp garam masala
- 1 red bell pepper, diced
- 1 ¼ cups coconut cream
- 1 tbsp cilantro, chopped

1. Preheat your oven to 400°F. Warm the olive oil in a skillet over medium heat. Season the tempeh with some salt. Fry the tempeh until browned on both sides, about 4 minutes.
2. Stir half of the garam masala into the tempeh until evenly mixed; turn the heat off. Transfer the tempeh with the spice into a baking dish.
3. Then, mix the bell pepper, coconut cream, cilantro, and remaining garam masala in a small bowl.
4. Pour the mixture over the tempeh and bake in the oven for 20 minutes or until golden brown on top. Garnish with cilantro and serve.

PER SERVING

Cal 595; Fat 50g; Carbs 20g; Protein 26g

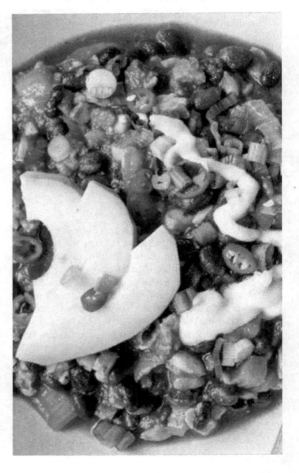

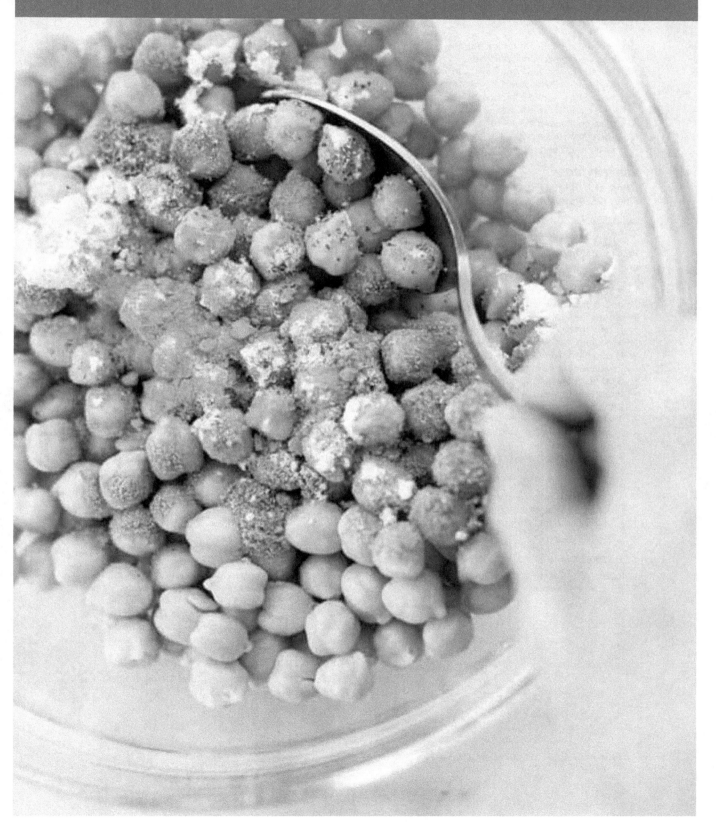

Chapter 11
Beans and Grains

Basic Beans

**Prep time: 8 hours to soak| Cook time:7 to 8 hours on low |
Makes 6 cups**

- 1 pound dried beans, any kind
- water

1. Rinse the beans, and pick out any broken ones or possible rocks or dirt particles.
2. Put the beans in a large bowl or in your slow cooker and cover with water. Let soak for a minimum of 8 hours, or overnight, at room temperature.
3. Drain and rinse the beans well. Put them in your slow cooker and cover with 2 inches of fresh water.
4. Cover the cooker and set to low. Cook for 7 to 8 hours, or until soft and cooked through. Drain and serve.

PER SERVING

Calories: 259; Total Fat: 0g; Total Carbs: 48g; Sugar: 2g; Fiber: 19g; Protein: 15g; Sodium: 0mg

Vegan Baked Navy Beans

Prep time: 15 minutes, plus 8 hours to soak| Cook time:7 to 8 hours on low | Serves 4

- 2 cups dried navy beans, soaked in water overnight, drained, and rinsed
- 6 cups vegetable broth
- ¼ cup dried cranberries
- 1 medium sweet onion, diced
- ½ cup all-natural ketchup (choose the one with the lowest amount of sugar)
- 3 tablespoons extra-virgin olive oil
- 2 tablespoons maple syrup
- 2 tablespoons molasses
- 1 tablespoon apple cider vinegar
- 1 teaspoon Dijon mustard
- 1 teaspoon sea salt
- ½ teaspoon garlic powder

1. In your slow cooker, combine the beans, broth, cranberries, onion, ketchup, olive oil, maple syrup, molasses, vinegar, mustard, salt, and garlic powder.
2. Cover the cooker and set to low. Cook for 7 to 8 hours and serve.

PER SERVING

Calories: 423; Total Fat: 11g; Total Carbs: 78g; Sugar: 25g; Fiber: 19g; Protein: 16g; Sodium: 1,731mg

Hatch Chile "Refried" Beans

Prep time: 15 minutes, plus 8 hours to soak|Cook time:6 to 8 hours on low | Serves 4

- 2 cups dried pinto beans, soaked in water overnight, drained, and rinsed
- 7 cups vegetable broth
- ½ medium onion, minced
- 1 (4-ounce) can Hatch green chiles
- 1 tablespoon freshly squeezed lime juice
- ½ teaspoon ground cumin
- ½ teaspoon garlic powder
- ½ teaspoon sea salt

1. In your slow cooker, combine the beans, broth, onion, chiles, lime juice, cumin, garlic powder, and salt.
2. Cover the cooker and set to low. Cook for 6 to 8 hours, until the beans are soft.
3. Using an immersion blender, mash the beans to your desired consistency before serving. If you don't own an immersion blender, mash the beans by hand with a fork or a potato masher.

PER SERVING

Calories: 218; Total Fat: 0g; Total Carbs: 49g; Sugar: 6g; Fiber: 18g; Protein: 16g; Sodium: 1,287mg

Indian Butter Chickpeas

Prep time: 15 minutes, plus 8 hours to soak| Cook time:6 to 8 hours on low | Serves 4

- 1 tablespoon coconut oil
- 1 medium onion, diced
- 1 pound dried chickpeas, soaked in water overnight, drained, and rinsed
- 2 cups full-fat coconut milk
- 1 (14.5-ounce) can crushed tomatoes
- 2 tablespoons almond butter
- 2 tablespoons curry powder
- 1½ teaspoons garlic powder
- 1 teaspoon ground ginger
- ½ teaspoon sea salt
- ½ teaspoon ground cumin
- ½ teaspoon chili powder

1. Coat the slow cooker with coconut oil.
2. Layer the onion along the bottom of the slow cooker.
3. Add the chickpeas, coconut milk, tomatoes, almond butter, curry powder, garlic powder, ginger, salt, cumin, and chili powder. Gently stir to ensure the spices are mixed into the liquid.
4. Cover the cooker and set to low. Cook for 6 to 8 hours, until the chickpeas are soft, and serve.

PER SERVING

Calories: 720; Total Fat: 30g; Total Carbs: 86g; Sugar: 9g; Fiber: 19g; Protein: 27g; Sodium: 440mg

Basic Quinoa

Prep time: 15 minutes of fewer| Cook time:4 to 6 hours on low | Serves 4

- 2 cups quinoa, rinsed well
- 4 cups vegetable broth

1. In your slow cooker, combine the quinoa and broth.
2. Cover the cooker and set to low. Cook for 4 to 6 hours. Fluff with a fork, cool, and serve.

PER SERVING

Calories: 335; Total Fat: 5g; Total Carbs: 61g; Sugar: 2g; Fiber: 7g; Protein: 12g; Sodium: 550mg

Mediterranean Quinoa with Peperoncini

Prep time: 15 minutes or fewer| Cook time:6 to 8 hours on low | Serves 4

- 1½ cups quinoa, rinsed well
- 3 cups vegetable broth
- ½ teaspoon sea salt
- ½ teaspoon garlic powder
- ¼ teaspoon dried oregano
- ¼ teaspoon dried basil leaves
- Freshly ground black pepper
- 3 cups arugula
- ½ cup diced tomatoes
- ⅓ cup sliced peperoncini
- ¼ cup freshly squeezed lemon juice
- 3 tablespoons extra-virgin olive oil

1. In your slow cooker, combine the quinoa, broth, salt, garlic powder, oregano, and basil, and season with pepper.
2. Cover the cooker and set to low. Cook for 6 to 8 hours.
3. In a large bowl, toss together the arugula, tomatoes, peperoncini, lemon juice, and olive oil.
4. When the quinoa is done, add it to the arugula salad, mix well, and serve.

PER SERVING

Calories: 359; Total Fat: 14g; Total Carbs: 50g; Sugar: 2g; Fiber: 6g; Protein: 10g; Sodium: 789mg

Coconutty Brown Rice

Prep time: 15 minutes, plus 8 hours to soak| Cook time:3 hours on high | Serves 4

- 2 cups brown rice, soaked in water overnight, drained, and rinsed
- 3 cups water
- 1½ cups full-fat coconut milk
- 1 teaspoon sea salt
- ½ teaspoon ground ginger
- Freshly ground black pepper

1. In your slow cooker, combine the rice, water, coconut milk, salt, and ginger. Season with pepper and stir to incorporate the spices.
2. Cover the cooker and set to high. Cook for 3 hours and serve.

PER SERVING

Calories: 479; Total Fat: 19g; Total Carbs: 73g; Sugar: 1g; Fiber: 4g; Protein: 9g; Sodium: 604mg

Herbed Harvest Rice

Prep time: 15 minutes, plus 8 hours to soak| Cook time:3 hours on high | Serves 4

- 2 cups brown rice, soaked in water overnight, drained, and rinsed
- ½ small onion, chopped
- 4 cups vegetable broth
- 2 tablespoons extra-virgin olive oil
- ½ teaspoon dried thyme leaves
- ½ teaspoon garlic powder
- ½ cup cooked sliced mushrooms
- ½ cup dried cranberries
- ½ cup toasted pecans

1. In your slow cooker, combine the rice, onion, broth, olive oil, thyme, and garlic powder. Stir well.
2. Cover the cooker and set to high. Cook for 3 hours.
3. Stir in the mushrooms, cranberries, and pecans, and serve.

PER SERVING

Calories: 546; Total Fat: 20g; Total Carbs: 88g; Sugar: 14g; Fiber: 7g; Protein: 10g; Sodium: 607mg

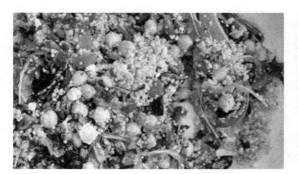

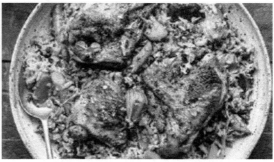

Spanish Rice

Prep time: 15 minutes or fewer | Cook time: 5 to 6 hours on low | Serves 4

- 2 cups white rice
- 2 cups vegetable broth
- 2 tablespoons extra-virgin olive oil
- 1 (14.5-ounce) can crushed tomatoes
- 1 (4-ounce) can Hatch green chiles
- ½ medium onion, diced
- 1 teaspoon sea salt
- ½ teaspoon ground cumin
- ½ teaspoon garlic powder
- ½ teaspoon chili powder
- ½ teaspoon dried oregano
- Freshly ground black pepper

1. In your slow cooker, combine the rice, broth, olive oil, tomatoes, chiles, onion, salt, cumin, garlic powder, chili powder, and oregano, and season with pepper.
2. Cover the cooker and set to low. Cook for 5 to 6 hours, fluff, and serve.

PER SERVING

Calories: 406; Total Fat: 7g; Total Carbs: 79g; Sugar: 5g; Fiber: 2g; Protein: 8g; Sodium: 1,058mg

Veggie "Fried" Quinoa

Prep time: 15 minutes or fewer | Cook time: 4 to 6 hours on low | Serves 4

- 2 cups quinoa, rinsed well
- 4 cups vegetable broth
- ¼ cup sliced carrots
- ¼ cup corn kernels
- ¼ cup green peas
- ¼ cup diced scallion
- 1 tablespoon sesame oil
- 1 teaspoon garlic powder
- 1 teaspoon sea salt
- Dash red pepper flakes

1. In your slow cooker, combine the quinoa, broth, carrots, corn, peas, scallion, sesame oil, garlic powder, salt, and red pepper flakes.
2. Cover the cooker and set to low. Cook for 4 to 6 hours, fluff, and serve.

PER SERVING

Calories: 387; Total Fat: 8g; Total Carbs: 65g; Sugar: 4g; Fiber: 8g; Protein: 13g; Sodium: 1,147mg

Bean & Rice Casserole

Prep time: 5 minutes | Cook time: 40 minutes | Serves 4

- 1 cup soaked black beans
- 2 cups water
- 2 tsp onion powder
- 2 tsp chili powder, optional
- 2 cups brown rice
- 6 oz tomato paste
- 1 tsp minced garlic
- 1 tsp sea salt

1. Combine all of the ingredients in your Instant Pot. Choose the "Manual" setting and seal the lid. Cook for 35 minutes on high pressure.
2. Once the cooking is complete, let the pressure release for 5 minutes. Then perform a quick pressure release. Serve hot.

PER SERVING

Cal 320; Fat 2g; Carbs 65g; Protein 6g

Chili Bean & Brown Rice Tortillas

Prep time: 5 minutes | Cook time: 50 minutes | Serves 4

- 1 cup brown rice
- Sea salt and pepper to taste
- 1 tbsp olive oil
- 1 red onion, chopped
- 1 green bell pepper, diced
- 2 garlic cloves, minced
- 1 tbsp chili powder
- 1 tsp cumin powder
- 1/8 tsp red chili flakes
- 1 (15 oz) can black beans
- 4 whole-wheat tortillas, warm
- 1 cup salsa
- 1 cup coconut cream

1. Add 2 cups of water and brown rice to a medium pot, season with some salt, and cook over medium heat until the water absorbs and the rice is tender, 15-20 minutes.
2. Heat the olive oil in a medium skillet over medium heat and sauté the onion, bell pepper, and garlic until softened and fragrant, 3 minutes.
3. Mix in the chili powder, cumin powder, red chili flakes, and season with salt and black pepper. Cook for 1 minute or until the food releases fragrance. Stir in the brown rice, black beans, and allow warming through, 3 minutes.
4. Lay the tortillas on a clean, flat surface and divide the rice mixture in the center of each. Top with salsa and coconut cream. Fold the sides and ends of the tortillas over the filling to secure. Serve.

PER SERVING

Cal 650; Fat 31g; Carbs 83g; Protein 9g

Zesty Rice Bowls with Tempeh

Prep time: 5 minutes | Cook time: 50 minutes | Serves 4

- 2 tbsp olive oil
- 1 ½ cups crumbled tempeh
- 1 tsp Creole seasoning
- 2 red bell peppers, sliced
- 1 cup brown rice
- 2 cups vegetable broth
- Sea salt to taste
- 1 lemon, zested and juiced
- 1 (8 oz) can black beans
- 2 chives, chopped
- 2 tbsp chopped parsley

1. Heat the olive oil in a medium pot and cook in the tempeh until golden brown, 5 minutes. Season with the Creole seasoning and stir in the bell peppers. Cook until the peppers slightly soften, 3 minutes.
2. Stir in the brown rice, vegetable broth, salt, and lemon zest.
3. Cover and cook until the rice is tender and all the liquid is absorbed, 15-25 minutes. Mix in the lemon juice, beans, and chives.
4. Allow warming for 3 to 5 minutes and dish the food. Garnish with the parsley and serve warm.

PER SERVING

Cal 540; Fat 16g; Carbs 76g; Protein 13g

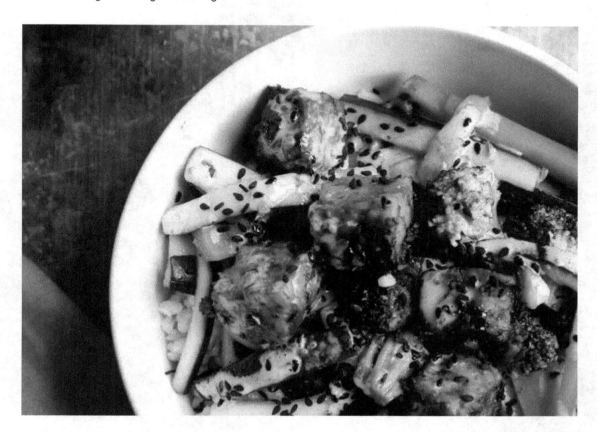

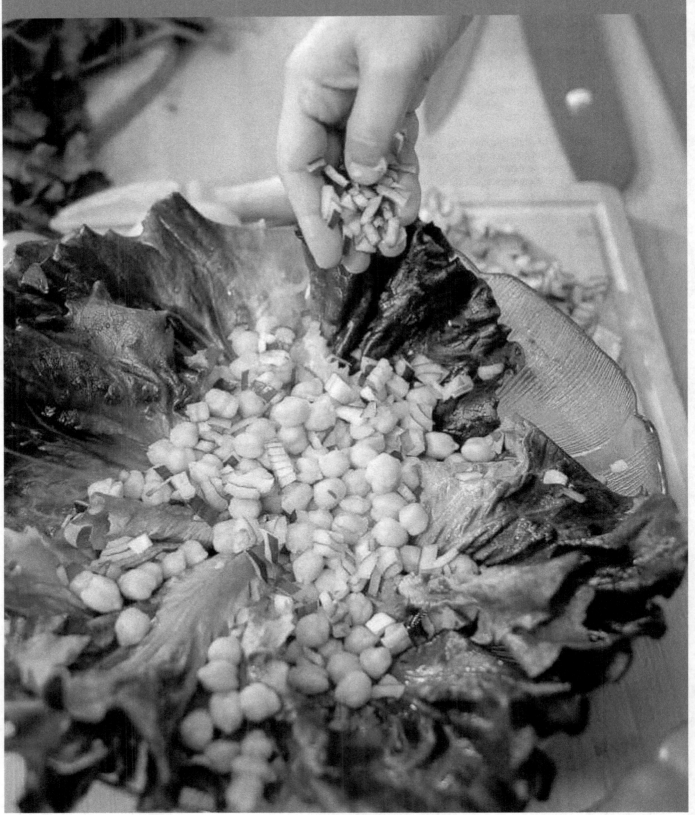

Spinach & Pomegranate Salad

Prep time: 5 minutes | Cook time: 10 minutes | Serves 4

- 2 tbsp extra-virgin olive oil
- 4 cups fresh baby spinach
- ¼ cup pomegranate seeds
- ¼ cup raspberry vinaigrette

1. Mix the spinach and walnuts in a bowl.
2. Sprinkle with olive oil and raspberry vinaigrette and toss to combine.

PER SERVING

Cal 500; Fat 49g; Carbs 10g; Protein 12g

Ginger Fruit Salad

Prep time: 5 minutes | Cook time: 10 minutes | Serves 4

- 1 nectarine, sliced
- ½ cup fresh blueberries
- ½ cup fresh raspberries
- ½ cup fresh strawberries
- 1 tbsp grated fresh ginger
- 1 orange, zested
- 1 orange, juiced

1. Mix the nectarine, blueberries, raspberries, strawberries, ginger, orange zest, and orange juice in a bowl. Serve.

PER SERVING

Cal 80; Fat 1g; Carbs 19g; Protein 2g

Quick Insalata Caprese

Prep time: 5 minutes | Cook time: 10 minutes | Serves 4

- 16 oz fresh mozzarella cheese, sliced
- 4 large tomatoes, sliced
- ¼ cup fresh basil leaves
- ¼ cup extra-virgin olive oil
- Sea salt and pepper to taste

1. On a salad platter, layer alternating slices of tomatoes and mozzarella.
2. Add a basil leaf between each slice. Season with olive oil, salt, and pepper. Serve right away.

PER SERVING

Cal 150; Fat 15g; Carbs 5g; Protein 1g

Maple Walnut & Pear Salad

Prep time: 5 minutes | Cook time: 10 minutes | Serves 4

- 4 cored pears, chopped
- ¼ cup walnuts, chopped
- 2 tbsp maple syrup
- 2 tbsp balsamic vinegar
- 2 tbsp extra-virgin olive oil

1. Mix the pears and walnuts in a bowl.
2. In another bowl, combine the maple syrup, balsamic vinegar, and olive oil, pour it over pears, and toss to coat. Serve immediately.

PER SERVING

Cal 280; Fat 14g; Carbs 43g; Protein 4g

Asparagus & Pasta Salad

Prep time: 5 minutes | Cook time: 30 Minutes | Serves 4

- 1 lb asparagus, sliced
- 2 cups arugula
- 1 cup basil sauce
- 1 tbsp olive oil
- 12 oz whole-wheat penne
- 2 scallions, sliced
- Sea salt and pepper to taste

1. Cook the pasta according to the package's instructions, then before cooking ends, about 2 minutes add the asparagus.
2. Strain them and place them back in the pot. Mix in basil sauce and olive oil. Let cool before combining the scallions, salt, and pepper. Serve right away.

PER SERVING

Cal 455; Fat 4g; Carbs 70g; Protein 13g

Chickpea & Celery Salad

Prep time: 5 minutes | Cook time: 5 minutes | Serves 4

- 1 (15.5-oz) can chickpeas
- 1 head fennel bulb, sliced
- ½ cup sliced red onion
- ½ cup celery leaves, chopped
- ¼ cup paleo mayonnaise
- Sea salt and pepper to taste

1. In a bowl, mash the chickpeas until chunky.
2. Stir in fennel bulb, onion, celery, mayonnaise, salt, and pepper. Serve.

PER SERVING

Cal 165; Fat 7g; Carbs 21g; Protein 7g

Traditional Lebanese Salad

Prep time: 5 minutes | Cook time: 25 minutes | Serves 4

- 1 cup cooked bulgur
- 1 cup boiling water
- Zest and juice of 1 lemon
- 1 garlic clove, pressed
- Sea salt to taste
- 1 tbsp olive oil
- ½ cucumber, sliced
- 1 tomato, sliced
- 1 cup fresh parsley, chopped
- ¼ cup fresh mint, chopped
- 2 scallions, chopped
- 4 tbsp sunflower seeds

1. Mix lemon juice, lemon zest, garlic, salt, and olive oil in a bowl. Stir in cucumber, tomato, parsley, mint, and scallions.
2. Toss to coat. Fluff the bulgur and stir it into the cucumber mix. Top with sunflower seeds and serve.

PER SERVING

Cal 140; Fat 8g; Carbs 14g; Protein 7g

Cucumber, Lettuce & Tomato Salad

Prep time: 5 minutes | Cook time: 15 minutes | Serves 4

- ½ cup halved pitted Kalamata olives
- ¾ cup olive oil
- ¼ cup white wine vinegar
- 2 tsp Dijon mustard
- 1 garlic clove
- 1 tbsp minced green onions
- ½ head romaine lettuce, torn
- ½ head iceberg lettuce, torn
- 1 (15.5-oz) can lentils
- 2 ripe tomatoes, chopped
- 1 peeled cucumber, diced
- 1 carrot, chopped
- 3 red radishes, chopped
- 2 tbsp chopped parsley
- 1 ripe avocado, chopped
- Sea salt and pepper to taste

1. Put the oil, vinegar, mustard, garlic, green onions, salt, and pepper in a food processor. Pulse until blended. Set aside.
2. In a bowl, place the lettuces, lentils, tomatoes, cucumber, carrot, olives, radishes, parsley, and avocado. Pour enough dressing over the salad and toss to coat.

PER SERVING

Cal 560; Fat 50g; Carbs 27g; Protein 8g

Tropical Salad

Prep time: 5 minutes | Cook time: 15 minutes | Serves 4

- 2 cups blanched snow peas, sliced
- ½ cup chopped roasted almonds
- ½ tsp minced garlic
- ½ tsp grated fresh ginger
- ¼ cup olive oil
- ¼ tsp crushed red pepper
- 3 tbsp rice vinegar
- 3 tbsp water
- 1 tsp low-sodium soy sauce
- ½ papaya, chopped
- 1 large carrot, shredded
- 1 peeled cucumber, sliced
- 1 shredded romaine lettuce
- Sea salt to taste

1. Combine garlic, ginger, olive oil, red pepper, vinegar, water, salt, and soy sauce in a bowl.
2. Add papaya, snow peas, cucumber slices, and carrot and toss to coat. Spread the lettuce on a plate. Top with salad and almonds.

PER SERVING

Cal 280; Fat 20g; Carbs 23g; Protein 1g

Italian Vegetable Relish

Prep time: 5 minutes | Cook time: 15 minutes | Serves 6

- ¼ cup sliced pimiento-stuffed green olives
- 1 carrot, sliced
- 1 red bell pepper, sliced
- 1 cup cauliflower florets
- 2 celery stalks, chopped
- ½ cup chopped red onion
- 1 garlic clove, minced
- 1 jalapeño pepper, chopped
- 3 tbsp white wine vinegar
- 1/3 cup olive oil
- Sea salt to taste

1. Combine the carrot, bell pepper, cauliflower, celery, and onion in a bowl. Add in salt and cold water. Cover and transfer to the fridge for 4-6 hours. Strain and wash the veggies. Remove to a bowl and mix in olives. Set aside.
2. In another bowl, mix the garlic, jalapeño pepper, vinegar, and olive oil. Pour over the veggies and toss to coat. Let chill in the fridge for at least 2 hours. Serve and enjoy!

PER SERVING

Cal 135; Fat 13g; Carbs 4g; Protein 1g

Mediterranean Pasta Salad

Prep time: 5 minutes | Cook time: 15 minutes | Serves 4

- ½ cup minced sun-dried tomatoes
- 2 roasted bell red peppers, chopped
- 8 oz whole-wheat pasta
- 1 (15.5-oz) can chickpeas
- ½ cup pitted black olives
- 1 (6-oz) jar dill pickles, sliced
- ½ cup frozen peas, thawed
- 1 tbsp capers
- 3 tsp dried chives
- ½ cup olive oil
- ¼ cup white wine vinegar
- ½ tsp dried basil
- 1 garlic clove, minced
- Sea salt and pepper to taste

1. Cook the pasta in salted water for 8-10 minutes until al dente. Drain and remove to a bowl. Stir in chickpeas, black olives, sun-dried tomatoes, dill pickles, roasted peppers, peas, capers, and chives.
2. In another bowl, whisk oil, white wine vinegar, basil, garlic, sugar, salt, and pepper. Pour over the pasta and toss to coat. Serve.

PER SERVING

Cal 590; Fat 32g; Carbs 67g; Protein 12g

Zucchini & Bell Pepper Salad with Beans

Prep time: 5 minutes | Cook time: 40 minutes | Serves 2

- 1 (14-oz) can cannellini beans
- 1 tbsp olive oil
- 2 tbsp balsamic vinegar
- 1 tsp minced fresh chives
- 1 garlic clove, minced
- 1 tbsp rosemary, chopped
- 1 tbsp oregano, chopped
- A pinch of sea salt
- 1 green bell pepper, sliced
- 1 zucchini, diced
- 2 carrots, diced

1. In a bowl, mix the olive oil, balsamic vinegar, chives, garlic, rosemary, oregano, and salt.
2. Stir in the beans, bell pepper, zucchini, and carrots. Serve and enjoy!

PER SERVING

Cal 150; Fat 8g; Carbs 1g; Protein 1g

Bulgur & Kale Salad

Prep time: 5 minutes | Cook time: 30 minutes | Serves 4

- ½ cup chopped green beans, steamed
- 1 avocado, peeled and pitted
- 1 tbsp fresh lemon juice
- 1 small garlic clove, pressed
- 1 scallion, chopped
- Sea salt to taste
- 8 large kale leaves, chopped
- 16 cherry tomatoes, halved
- 1 red bell pepper, chopped
- 2 scallions, chopped
- 2 cups cooked bulgur

1. In a food processor, place the avocado, lemon juice, garlic, scallion, salt, and ¼ cup water. Blend until smooth.
2. Set aside the dressing. Put kale, green beans, cherry tomatoes, bell pepper, scallions, and bulgur in a serving bowl. Add in the dressing and toss to coat. Serve.

PER SERVING

Cal 200; Fat 8g; Carbs 30.3g; Protein 5g

Minty Eggplant Salad

Prep time: 5 minutes | Cook time: 45 minutes | Serves 2

- 1 lemon, half zested and juiced, half cut into wedges
- 1 tsp olive oil
- 1 eggplant, chopped
- ½ tsp ground cumin
- ½ tsp ground ginger
- ¼ tsp turmeric
- ¼ tsp ground nutmeg
- Sea salt to taste
- 2 tbsp capers
- 1 tbsp chopped green olives
- 1 garlic clove, pressed
- 2 tbsp fresh mint, chopped
- 2 cups watercress, chopped

1. In a skillet over medium heat, warm the oil. Place the eggplant and cook for 5 minutes. Add in cumin, ginger, turmeric, nutmeg, and salt. Cook for another 10 minutes.
2. Stir in lemon zest, lemon juice, capers, olives, garlic, and mint. Cook for 1-2 minutes more. Place some watercress on each plate and top with the eggplant mixture. Serve.

PER SERVING

Cal 110; Fat 3g; Carbs 20g; Protein 44g

Cashew & Raisin Salad

Prep time: 5 minutes | Cook time: 15 minutes | Serves 4

- 3 cups haricots verts, trimmed and chopped
- 2 carrots, sliced
- 3 cups shredded cabbage
- 1/3 cup golden raisins
- ¼ cup roasted cashew
- 1 garlic clove, minced
- 1 medium shallot, chopped
- 1½ tsp grated fresh ginger
- 1/3 cup creamy peanut butter
- 2 tsp low-sodium soy sauce
- 2 tbsp fresh lemon juice
- Sea salt to taste
- ⅛ tsp ground cayenne
- ¾ cup coconut milk

1. Place the haricots verts, carrots, and cabbage in a pot with water and steam for 5 minutes. Drain and transfer to a bowl. Add in raisins and cashew. Let cool.
2. In a food processor, put the garlic, shallot, and ginger. Pulse until puréed. Add in peanut butter, soy sauce, lemon juice, salt, cayenne pepper. Blitz until smooth.
3. Stir in coconut milk. Sprinkle the salad with the dressing and toss to coat.

PER SERVING

Cal 410; Fat 31g; Carbs 30g; Protein 40g

Lettuce & Tomato Salad with Quinoa

Prep time: 5 minutes | Cook time: 25 minutes | Serves 4

- 1 cup quinoa, rinsed
- ⅓ cup white wine vinegar
- 2 tbsp extra-virgin olive oil
- 1 tbsp chopped fresh dill
- Sea salt and pepper to taste
- 2 cups sliced sweet onions
- 2 tomatoes, sliced
- 4 cups shredded lettuce

1. Place the quinoa in a pot with 2 cups of salted water. Bring to a boil. Lower the heat and simmer covered for 15 minutes. Turn the heat off and let sit for 5 minutes. Using a fork, fluff the quinoa and set aside.
2. In a small bowl, whisk the vinegar, olive oil, dill, salt, and pepper; set aside. In a serving plate, combine onions, tomatoes, quinoa, and lettuce. Pour in the dressing and toss to coat.

PER SERVING

Cal 380; Fat 11g; Carbs 58g; Protein 12g

Bell Pepper & Quinoa Salad

Prep time: 5 minutes | Cook time: 15 minutes | Serves 4

- 2 cups cooked quinoa
- ½ red onion, diced
- 1 red bell pepper, diced
- 1 orange bell pepper, diced
- 1 carrot, diced
- ¼ cup olive oil
- 2 tbsp rice vinegar
- 1 tsp low-sodium soy sauce
- 1 garlic clove, minced
- 1 tbsp grated fresh ginger
- Sea salt and pepper to taste

1. Combine the quinoa, onion, bell peppers, and carrots in a bowl.
2. In another bowl, mix the olive oil, rice vinegar, soy sauce, garlic, ginger, salt, and pepper. Pour over the quinoa and toss to coat. Serve and enjoy!

PER SERVING

Cal 270; Fat 16g; Carbs 28g; Protein 6g

Radish & Cabbage Ginger Salad

Prep time: 5 minutes | Cook time: 15 minutes | Serves 4

- 8 oz napa cabbage, cut crosswise into strips
- 2 tbsp chopped roasted hazelnuts
- 1 cup grated carrots
- 1 cup sliced radishes
- 2 green onions, minced
- 2 tbsp chopped parsley
- 2 tbsp rice vinegar
- 2 tsp olive oil
- 1 tsp low-sodium soy sauce
- 1 tsp grated fresh ginger
- ½ tsp dry mustard
- Sea salt and pepper to taste

1. Place the cabbage, carrot, radishes, green onions, and parsley in a bowl, stir to combine.
2. In another bowl, mix vinegar, olive oil, soy sauce, ginger, mustard, salt, and pepper. Pour over the slaw and toss to coat. Place in the fridge for 2 hours. Serve topped with hazelnuts.

PER SERVING

Cal 80; Fat 6g; Carbs 6g; Protein 10g

Easy Pineapple & Jicama Salad

Prep time: 5 minutes | Cook time: 15 minutes | Serves 6

- 1 jicama, peeled and grated
- 1 peeled pineapple, sliced
- ¼ cup non-dairy milk
- 2 tbsp fresh basil, chopped
- 1 large scallion, chopped
- Sea salt to taste
- 1½ tbsp tahini
- arugula for serving
- Chopped cashews

1. Place jicama in a bowl. In a food processor, put the pineapple and enough milk. Blitz until puréed.
2. Add in basil, scallions, tahini, and salt. Pour over the jicama and cover. Transfer to the fridge and marinate for 1 hour.
3. Place a bed of arugula on a plate and top with the salad. Serve garnished with cashews.

PER SERVING

Cal 175; Fat 5g; Carbs 33g; Protein 2g

Broccoli & Mango Rice Salad

Prep time: 5 minutes | Cook time: 25 minutes | Serves 4

- 3 cups broccoli florets, blanched
- 1/3 cup roasted almonds, chopped
- ½ cup brown rice, rinsed
- 1 mango, chopped
- 1 red bell pepper, chopped
- 1 jalapeño, minced
- 1 tsp grated fresh ginger
- 2 tbsp fresh lemon juice
- 3 tbsp grapeseed oil

1. Place the rice in a bowl with salted water and cook for 18-20 minutes. Remove to a bowl.
2. Stir in broccoli, mango, bell pepper, and chili. In another bowl, mix the ginger, lemon juice, and oil. Pour over the rice and toss to combine. Top with almonds. Serve and enjoy!

PER SERVING

Cal 290; Fat 15g; Carbs 35g; Protein 1g

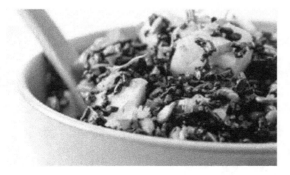

Mom's Caesar Salad

Prep time: 5 minutes | Cook time: 10 minutes | Serves 4

- ½ cup cashews
- ½ cup water
- 3 tbsp olive oil
- Juice of ½ lime
- 1 tbsp white miso paste
- 1 tsp low-sodium soy sauce
- 1 tsp Dijon mustard
- 1 tsp garlic powder
- Sea salt and pepper to taste
- 2 heads romaine lettuce, torn
- 2 tsp capers
- 1 cup cherry tomatoes, halved
- 4 oz shaved Parmesan cheese
- Whole-what bread croutons

1. In a blender, put cashews, water, olive oil, lime juice, miso paste, soy sauce, mustard, garlic powder, salt, and pepper. Blend until smooth.
2. Mix the lettuce with half of the dressing in a bowl. Add capers, tomatoes, and Parmesan cheese. Serve topped with croutons.

PER SERVING

Cal 415; Fat 28g; Carbs 30g; Protein 17g

Fantastic Green Salad

Prep time: 5 minutes | Cook time: 10 minutes | Serves 4

- 1 head Iceberg lettuce
- 8 asparagus, chopped
- 2 seedless cucumbers, sliced
- 1 zucchini, cut into ribbons
- 1 carrot, cut into ribbons
- 1 avocado, sliced
- ½ cup green dressing
- 2 scallions, thinly sliced

1. Share the lettuce into 4 bowls and add in some asparagus, cucumber, zucchini, carrot, and avocado.
2. Sprinkle each bowl with 2 tbsp of dressing. Serve topped with scallions.

PER SERVING

Cal 255; Fat 21g; Carbs 15g; Protein 4g

Chickpea & Quinoa Salad with Capers

Prep time: 5 minutes | Cook time: 25 minutes | Serves 4

- 1 cup quinoa, rinsed
- 1 (15.5-oz) can chickpeas
- 1 cup cherry tomatoes, halved
- 2 green onions, minced
- ½ peeled cucumber, chopped
- ¼ cup capers
- 2 tbsp toasted pine nuts
- 1 medium shallot, sliced
- 1 garlic clove, chopped
- 1 tsp Dijon mustard
- 2 tbsp white wine vinegar
- ¼ cup olive oil
- Sea salt and pepper to taste

1. Boil salted water in a pot over medium heat. Add in quinoa, lower the heat and simmer for 15 minutes. Remove to a bowl. Stir in chickpeas, tomatoes, green onions, cucumber, capers, and pine nuts. Set aside.
2. In a food processor, put the shallot, garlic, mustard, vinegar, oil, salt, and pepper. Pulse until blend. Pour over the salad and toss to coat. Serve immediately.

PER SERVING

Cal 410; Fat 21g; Carbs 46g; Protein 12g

Apple & Spinach Salad with Walnuts

Prep time: 5 minutes | Cook time: 20 minutes | Serves 4

- ¼ cup tahini
- 2 tbsp Dijon mustard
- 1 tbsp maple syrup
- 1 tbsp lemon juice
- ½ cup chopped walnuts
- 2 tsp low-sodium soy sauce
- 1 lb baby spinach
- 1 cored green apple, sliced
- Sea salt to taste

1. Preheat your oven to 360°F. Line with parchment paper a baking sheet. In a bowl, mix the tahini, mustard, 1 tbsp maple syrup, lemon juice, and salt. Set aside the dressing.
2. In another bowl, combine the walnuts, soy sauce, and the remaining maple syrup. Spread evenly on the baking sheet and bake for 5 minutes, shaking once until crunchy. Allow cooling for 3 minutes.
3. Combine the spinach and apples in a bowl. Pour over the dressing and toss to coat. Serve garnished with the walnut crunch.

PER SERVING

Cal 250; Fat 15g; Carbs 26g; Protein 8g

Apple & Arugula Salad with Walnuts

Prep time: 5 minutes | Cook time: 20 minutes | Serves 4

- ¼ cup chopped walnuts
- 10 oz arugula
- 1 apple, thinly sliced
- 1 tbsp finely minced shallot
- 2 tbsp champagne vinegar
- 2 tbsp olive oil
- Sea salt and pepper to taste
- ¼ tsp English mustard

1. Preheat your oven to 360°F. In a baking sheet, spread the walnuts and toast for 6 minutes. Let cool.
2. In a bowl, combine the walnuts, arugula, and apple. In another bowl, mix the shallot, vinegar, olive oil, salt, pepper, and mustard. Pour over the salad and toss to coat. Serve.

PER SERVING

Cal 140; Fat 11g; Carbs 10g; Protein 3g

Bean & Roasted Parsnip Salad

Prep time: 5 minutes | Cook time: 40 minutes | Serves 3

- 1 (15-oz) can cannellini beans
- 4 parsnips, sliced
- 2 tsp olive oil
- ½ tsp ground cinnamon
- Sea salt to taste
- 3 cups chopped spinach
- 2 tsp pomegranate seeds
- 2 tsp sunflower seeds
- ¼ cup raspberry vinaigrette

1. Preheat your oven to 390°F. In a bowl, combine parsnips, olive oil, cinnamon, and salt. Spread on a baking tray and roast for 15 minutes. Flip the parsnips and add the beans. Roast for another 15 minutes. Allow cooling.
2. Divide the spinach among plates and place the pomegranate seeds, sunflower seeds, and roasted parsnips and beans. Sprinkle with raspberry vinaigrette and serve.

PER SERVING

Cal 300; Fat 12g; Carbs 45g; Protein 8g

Green Mango Slaw With Cashews

Prep time: 5 minutes | Cook time: 35 minutes| Serves 4

FOR THE DRESSING

- 1 cup canned lite coconut milk
- 2 tablespoons freshly squeezed lime juice
- 2 tablespoons almond butter
- 1 teaspoon grated fresh ginger
- 1 teaspoon mild curry powder

FOR THE SALAD

- 3 cups fresh spinach
- 2 green mangos, peeled, pitted, and julienned
- 1 jicama, shredded
- 1 carrot, shredded, or ½ cup preshredded packaged carrots
- 1 scallion, white and green parts, julienned
- 2 tablespoons chopped fresh cilantro
- ¼ cup chopped cashews, for garnish

TO MAKE THE DRESSING

- In a small bowl, whisk the coconut milk, lime juice, almond butter, ginger, and curry powder until well blended. Set it aside.

TO MAKE THE SALAD

1. In a large bowl, toss together the spinach, mangos, jicama, carrot, and scallion.
2. Add the dressing and toss to coat.
3. Serve topped with the cilantro and cashews.

PER SERVING

Calories: 415; Total fat: 24g; Saturated fat: 14g; Carbohydrates: 50g; Fiber: 14g; Protein: 8g

Watermelon-Cucumber Salad

Prep time: 5 minutes | Cook time: 25 minutes| Serves 4

FOR THE DRESSING

- ½ cup olive oil
- ¼ cup apple cider vinegar
- 2 tablespoons raw honey
- 1 teaspoon freshly grated lemon zest (optional)
- Pinch sea salt

FOR THE SALAD

- 4 cups (½-inch) watermelon cubes
- 1 English cucumber, cut into ½-inch cubes
- 1 cup halved snow peas
- 1 scallion, white and green parts, chopped
- 2 cups shredded kale
- 1 tablespoon chopped fresh cilantro

TO MAKE THE DRESSING

In a small bowl, whisk the olive oil, cider vinegar, honey, and lemon zest (if using). Season with sea salt and set it aside.

TO MAKE THE SALAD

1. In a large bowl, toss together the watermelon, cucumber, snow peas, scallion, and dressing.
2. Divide the kale among four plates and top with the water-melon mixture.
3. Serve garnished with the cilantro.

PER SERVING

Calories: 353; Total fat: 26g; Saturated fat: 4g; Carbohydrates: 30g; Fiber: 3g; Protein: 4g

Massaged Swiss Chard Salad with Chopped Egg

Prep time: 5 minutes | Cook time: 25 minutes| Serves 4

FOR THE DRESSING

- ¼ cup olive oil
- 3 tablespoons freshly squeezed lemon juice
- 2 teaspoons raw honey
- 1 teaspoon Dijon mustard
- Sea salt

FOR THE SALAD

- 5 cups chopped Swiss chard
- 3 large hardboiled eggs, peeled and chopped
- 1 English cucumber, diced
- ½ cup sliced radishes
- ½ cup chopped pecans

TO MAKE THE DRESSING

In a small bowl, whisk the olive oil, lemon juice, honey, and mustard. Season with salt and set it aside.

TO MAKE THE SALAD

1. In a large bowl, toss the Swiss chard and dressing together for about 4 minutes, or until the greens start to soften. Divide the greens evenly among four plates.
2. Top each salad with egg, cucumber, radishes, and pecans.

PER SERVING

Calories: 241; Total fat: 21g; Saturated fat: 3g; Carbohydrates: 9g; Fiber: 2g; Protein: 7g

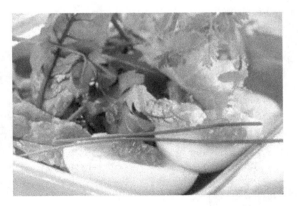

Coconut Fruit Salad

Prep time: 5 minutes | Cook time: 25 minutes| Serves 4

FOR THE DRESSING

¾ cup canned lite coconut milk
2 tablespoons almond butter
2 tablespoons freshly squeezed lime juice

FOR THE SALAD

6 cups mixed greens
½ pineapple, peeled, cored, and diced, or 3 cups precut packaged pineapple
1 mango, peeled, pitted, and diced, or 2 cups frozen chunks, thawed
1 cup quartered fresh strawberries
1 cup (1-inch) green bean pieces
½ cup shredded unsweetened coconut
1 tablespoon chopped fresh basil

TO MAKE THE DRESSING

In a small bowl, whisk the coconut milk, almond butter, and lime juice until smooth. Set it aside.

TO MAKE THE SALAD

1. In a large bowl, toss the mixed greens with three-fourths of the dressing. Arrange the salad on four plates.
2. In the same bowl, toss the pineapple, mango, strawberries, and green beans with the remaining fourth of the dressing.
3. Top each salad with the fruit and vegetable mixture and serve garnished with the coconut and basil.

PER SERVING

Calories: 311; Total fat: 19g; Saturated fat: 13g; Carbohydrates: 36g; Fiber: 7g; Protein: 5g

Grapefruit-Avocado Salad

Prep time: 5 minutes | Cook time: 25 minutes| Serves 4

FOR THE DRESSING

- ½ avocado, peeled and pitted
- ¼ cup freshly squeezed lemon juice
- 2 tablespoons raw honey
- Pinch sea salt
- Water, for thinning the dressing

FOR THE SALAD

- 4 cups fresh spinach
- 1 Ruby Red grapefruit, peeled, sectioned, and cut into chunks
- ¼ cup sliced radishes
- ¼ cup roasted sunflower seeds
- ¼ cup dried cranberries

TO MAKE THE DRESSING

1. 1. In a blender, combine the avocado, lemon juice, honey, and sea salt. Pulse until very smooth.
2. 2. Add enough water to reach your desired consistency and set the dressing aside.

TO MAKE THE SALAD

3. In a large bowl toss the spinach with half the dressing. Divide the dressed spinach among four plates.
4. Top each with grapefruit, radishes, sunflower seeds, and cranberries.
5. Drizzle the remaining half of the dressing over the salads and serve.

PER SERVING

Calories: 126; Total fat: 7g; Saturated fat: 1g; Carbohydrates: 16g; Fiber: 3g; Protein: 2g

Shredded Root Vegetable Salad

Prep time: 5 minutes | Cook time: 25 minutes| Serves 4

FOR THE DRESSING

- ¼ cup olive oil
- 3 tablespoons pure maple syrup
- 2 tablespoons apple cider vinegar
- 1 teaspoon grated fresh ginger
- Sea salt

FOR THE SLAW

- 1 jicama, or 2 parsnips, peeled and shredded
- 2 carrots, shredded, or 1 cup preshredded packaged carrots
- ½ celeriac, peeled and shredded
- ¼ fennel bulb, shredded
- 5 radishes, shredded
- 2 scallions, white and green parts, peeled and thinly sliced
- ½ cup pumpkin seeds, roasted

TO MAKE THE DRESSING

In a small bowl, whisk the olive oil, maple syrup, cider vinegar, and ginger until well blended. Season with sea salt and set it aside.

TO MAKE THE SLAW

1. In a large bowl, toss together the jicama, carrots, celeriac, fennel, radishes, and scallions.
2. Add the dressing and toss to coat.
3. Top the slaw with the pumpkin seeds and serve.

PER SERVING

Calories: 343; Total fat: 21g; Saturated fat: 3g; Carbohydrates: 36g; Fiber: 11g; Protein: 7g

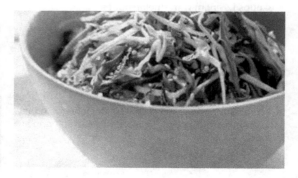

Artichoke-Almond Salad

Prep time: 5 minutes | Cook time: 25 minutes| Serves 4

- 2 cups cooked quinoa
- 2 (15-ounce) cans water-packed artichoke hearts, drained
- 1 cup chopped kale
- ½ cup chopped red onion
- ½ cup chopped almonds
- 3 tablespoons finely chopped fresh parsley
- Juice of 1 lemon (or 3 tablespoons)
- Zest of 1 lemon (optional)
- 2 tablespoons olive oil
- 1 tablespoon balsamic vinegar
- 1 teaspoon bottled minced garlic
- Sea salt

1. In a large bowl, toss together the quinoa, artichoke hearts, kale, red onion, almonds, parsley, lemon juice, lemon zest (if using), olive oil, balsamic vinegar, and garlic until well mixed.
2. Season with sea salt and serve.

PER SERVING

Calories: 402; Total fat: 16g; Saturated fat: 2g; Carbohydrates: 56g; Fiber: 17g; Protein: 16g

Mint Melon Salad

Prep time: 5 minutes | Cook time: 25 minutes| Serves 4

FOR THE DRESSING

- 3 tablespoons olive oil
- 2 tablespoons red wine vinegar
- Sea salt

FOR THE SALAD

- 1 honeydew melon, rind removed, flesh cut into 1-inch cubes
- ½ cantaloupe, rind removed, flesh cut into 1-inch cubes
- 3 stalks celery, sliced, or about 1 to 1½ cups precut packaged celery
- ½ red onion, thinly sliced
- ¼ cup chopped fresh mint

TO MAKE THE DRESSING

In a small bowl, whisk the olive oil and red wine vinegar. Season with sea salt and set it aside.

TO MAKE THE SALAD

1. In a large bowl, combine the honeydew, cantaloupe, celery, red onion, and mint.
2. Add the dressing and toss to combine.

PER SERVING

Calories: 223; Total fat: 11g; Saturated fat: 2g; Carbohydrates: 32g; Fiber: 4g; Protein: 2g

Broccoli Salad With Rainier Cherry Dressing

Prep time: 5 minutes | Cook time: 25 minutes| Serves 4

FOR THE DRESSING

- ½ cup Rainier cherries, pitted
- ¼ cup olive oil
- 2 tablespoons freshly squeezed lemon juice
- 2 tablespoons raw honey
- 1 teaspoon chopped fresh basil
- Pinch sea salt

FOR THE SALAD

- 4 cups broccoli florets, lightly blanched
- 2 cups mixed greens
- 1 cup snow peas
- ½ English cucumber, quartered lengthwise and sliced
- ½ red onion, thinly sliced

TO MAKE THE DRESSING

In a blender, combine the cherries, olive oil, lemon juice, honey, and basil. Pulse until smooth. Season with sea salt and set it aside.

TO MAKE THE SALAD

1. In a large bowl, toss the broccoli, greens, snow peas, cucumber, and red onion with the dressing to coat.

PER SERVING

Calories: 189; Total fat: 13g; Saturated fat: 2g; Carbohydrates: 18g; Fiber: 3g; Protein: 3g

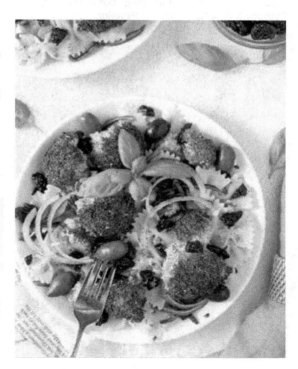

Turkey-Pecan Salad

Prep time: 5 minutes | Cook time: 25 minutes | Serves 4

FOR THE DRESSING

- ¼ cup olive oil
- 2 tablespoons balsamic vinegar
- 2 teaspoons whole-grain Dijon mustard
- 1 teaspoon chopped fresh thyme
- Sea salt

FOR THE SALAD

- 4 cups mixed greens
- 1 cup arugula
- ½ red onion, thinly sliced
- 16 ounces cooked turkey breast, chopped
- 3 apricots, pitted and each fruit cut into 8 pieces
- ½ cup chopped pecans

TO MAKE THE DRESSING

In a small bowl, whisk the olive oil, balsamic vinegar, mustard, and thyme. Season with sea salt and set it aside.

TO MAKE THE SALAD

1. In a large bowl, toss together the mixed greens, arugula, and red onion with three-fourths of the dressing. Arrange the dressed salad on a serving platter.
2. Top the greens with the turkey, apricots, and pecans.
3. Drizzle with the remaining fourth of the dressing and serve.

PER SERVING

Calories: 305; Total fat: 20g; Saturated fat: 3g; Carbohydrates: 12g; Fiber: 2g; Protein: 21g

Chickpea and Kale Salad

Prep time: 5 minutes | Cook time: 25 minutes | Serves 4

- 1 large bunch kale, thoroughly washed, stemmed, and cut into thin strips
- 2 teaspoons freshly squeezed lemon juice
- 2 tablespoons extra-virgin olive oil, divided
- ¾ teaspoon sea salt, divided
- 2 cups cooked chickpeas (about 1 [14-oz] can)
- 1 teaspoon sweet paprika
- 1 avocado, chopped (optional)

1. In a large bowl, combine the kale, lemon juice, 1 tablespoon of olive oil, and ¼ teaspoon of salt.
2. With your hands, massage the kale for 5 minutes, or until it starts to wilt and becomes bright green and shiny.
3. To a skillet set over medium-low heat, add the remaining 1 tablespoon of olive oil.
4. Stir in the chickpeas, paprika, and remaining ½ teaspoon of salt. Cook for about 15 minutes, or until warm. The chickpeas might start to crisp in spots.
5. Pour the chickpeas over the kale. Toss well. Add the avocado (if using).
6. Serve immediately.

PER SERVING

Calories: 359; Total Fat: 20g; Total Carbohydrates: 35g; Sugar: 1g; Fiber: 10g; Protein: 13g; Sodium: 497mg

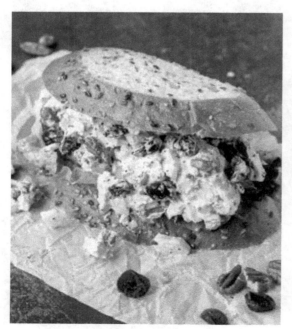

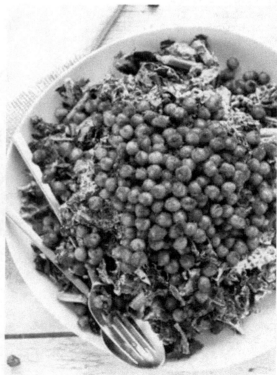

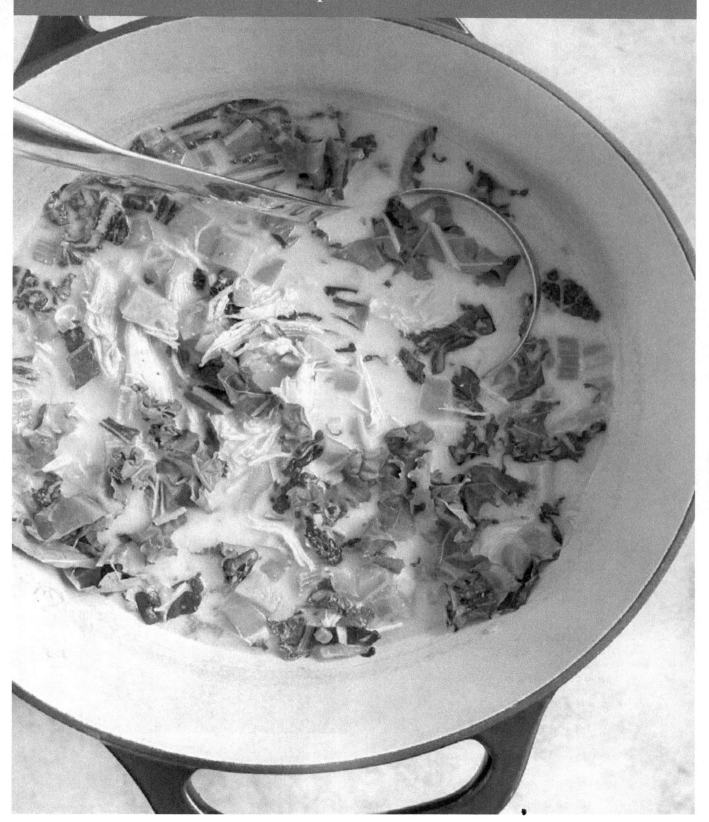

Lime Lentil Soup

Prep time: 5 minutes | Cook time: 35 minutes | Serves 2

- 1 tsp olive oil
- 1 onion, chopped
- 6 garlic cloves, minced
- 1 tsp chili powder
- ½ tsp ground cinnamon
- Sea salt to taste
- 1 cup yellow lentils
- 1 cup canned diced tomatoes
- 1 celery stalk, chopped
- 10 oz chopped collard greens

1. Heat oil in a pot over medium heat. Place onion and garlic and cook for 5 minutes. Stir in chili powder, celery, cinnamon, and salt.
2. Pour in lentils, tomatoes and juices, and 2 cups of water. Bring to a boil, then lower the heat and simmer for 15 minutes. Stir in collard greens. Cook for an additional 5 minutes. Serve in bowls and enjoy!

PER SERVING

Cal 155; Fat 3g; Carbs 29g; Protein 7g

Spinach, Rice & Bean Soup

Prep time: 5 minutes | Cook time: 45 minutes | Serves 6

- 6 cups baby spinach
- 2 tbsp extra-virgin olive oil
- 1 onion, chopped
- 2 garlic cloves, minced
- 15 oz canned black-eyed peas
- 6 cups vegetable broth
- Sea salt and pepper to taste
- ½ cup brown rice

1. Heat oil in a pot over medium heat. Place the onion and garlic and sauté for 3 minutes.
2. Pour in broth and season with salt and pepper. Bring to a boil, then lower the heat and stir in rice. Simmer for 15 minutes. Stir in peas and spinach and cook for another 5 minutes. Serve warm.

PER SERVING

Cal 200; Fat 5g; Carbs 32g; Protein 1g

Autumn Butternut Squash Soup

Prep time: 5 minutes | Cook time: 30 minutes | Serves 5

- 2 tbsp extra-virgin olive oil
- 2 lb butternut squash, cubed
- 1 red bell pepper, chopped
- 1 leek, chopped
- 3 garlic cloves, minced
- 2 celery stalks, chopped
- 4 cups vegetable broth
- 1 cup coconut yogurt

1. Heat the olive oil in a pot over medium heat. Add the red bell pepper, leek, garlic, and celery and sauté for 5 minutes until tender.
2. Pour in the broth and butternut squash and bring to a boil. Lower the heat and simmer for 20 minutes. Puree the soup with a stick blender until smooth.
3. Divide the soup between bowls and top with 1 tbsp of coconut yogurt each one. Serve and enjoy!

PER SERVING

Cal 225; Fat 17g; Carbs 19g; Protein 3g

Daikon & Sweet Potato Soup

Prep time: 5 minutes | Cook time: 40 minutes | Serves 6

- 6 cups water
- 2 tsp olive oil
- 1 chopped onion
- 3 garlic cloves, minced
- 1 tbsp thyme
- 2 tsp paprika
- 2 cups chopped daikon
- 2 cups diced sweet potatoes
- 2 cups chopped parsnips
- ½ tsp sea salt
- 1 cup fresh mint, chopped
- ½ avocado
- 2 tbsp balsamic vinegar
- 2 tbsp pumpkin seeds

1. Heat the oil in a pot and place onion and garlic. Sauté for 3 minutes. Add in thyme, paprika, daikon, sweet potato, parsnips, water, and salt.
2. Bring to a boil and cook for 30 minutes. Remove the soup to a food processor and add in balsamic vinegar; purée until smooth. Top with mint and pumpkin seeds to serve.

PER SERVING

Cal 150; Fat 6g; Carbs 24g; Protein 22g

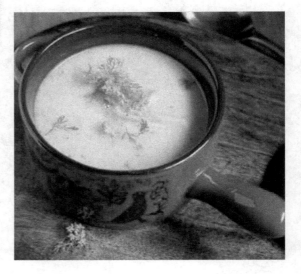

Italian Bean Soup

Prep time: 5 minutes | Cook time: 1 hour 25 minutes | Serves 6

- 3 tbsp extra-virgin olive oil
- 2 celery stalks, chopped
- 2 carrots, chopped
- 3 shallots, chopped
- 3 garlic cloves, minced
- ½ cup brown rice
- 6 cups vegetable broth
- 1 (14-oz) can diced tomatoes
- 2 bay leaves
- Sea salt and pepper to taste
- 2 (15.5-oz) cans white beans
- ¼ cup chopped basil

1. Heat oil in a pot over medium heat. Place celery, carrots, shallots, and garlic and cook for 5 minutes.
2. Add in brown rice, broth, tomatoes, bay leaves, salt, and pepper. Bring to a boil, then lower the heat and simmer uncovered for 20 minutes.
3. Stir in beans and basil and cook for 5 minutes. Discard bay leaves. Sprinkle with basil and serve.

PER SERVING

Cal 180; Fat 8g; Carbs 25g; Protein 2g

Gingered Broccoli Soup

Prep time: 5 minutes | Cook time: 50 minutes | Serves 4

- 1 onion, chopped
- 1 tbsp minced fresh ginger
- 2 tsp olive oil
- 2 carrots, chopped
- 10 oz broccoli florets
- 1 cup coconut milk
- 3 cups vegetable broth
- ½ tsp turmeric
- Sea salt and pepper to taste

1. In a pot over medium heat, place the onion, ginger, and olive oil, cook for 4 minutes.
2. Add in carrots, broccoli, broth, turmeric, pepper, and salt. Bring to a boil and cook for 15 minutes. Transfer the soup to a food processor and blend until smooth. Stir in coconut milk and serve.

PER SERVING

Cal 200; Fat 17g; Carbs 12g; Protein 3g

Celery Butternut Squash Soup

Prep time: 5 minutes | Cook time: 30 minutes | Serves 6

- 2 tbsp extra-virgin olive oil
- 1 onion, chopped
- 1 celery stalk, chopped
- ½ tsp ground allspice
- 1 carrot, chopped
- 1 lb butternut squash, cubed
- 6 cups vegetable broth
- Sea salt to taste
- 2 tbsp fresh orange juice

1. Heat the oil in a pot over medium heat. Place in onion and celery and sauté for 5 minutes until tender.
2. Add in allspice, carrot, squash, broth, and salt. Cook for 20 minutes. Stir in orange juice. Using an immersion blender, blitz the soup until purée. Serve immediately.

PER SERVING

Cal 95; Fat 5g; Carbs 14g; Protein 1g

Coconut & Tofu Soup

Prep time: 5 minutes | Cook time: 30 minutes | Serves 4

- 1 cup shiitake mushrooms, sliced
- 2 tbsp extra-virgin olive oil
- 1 onion, chopped
- 2 tbsp minced fresh ginger
- 2 tsp low-sodium soy sauce
- 1 tbsp pure date sugar
- 1 tsp chili paste
- 2 cups light vegetable broth
- 8 oz extra-firm tofu, cubed
- 2 (13.5-oz) cans coconut milk
- 1 tbsp fresh lime juice

1. Heat the oil in a pot over medium heat. Place in onion and ginger and sauté for 3 minutes until softened. Add in soy sauce, mushrooms, sugar, and chili paste. Stir in broth.
2. Bring to a boil, then lower the heat and simmer for 15 minutes. Strain the liquid and discard solids. Return the broth to the pot. Stir in tofu, coconut milk, and lime juice. Cook for 5 minutes. Serve and enjoy!

PER SERVING

Cal 630; Fat 60g; Carbs 22g; Protein 8g

Garlic Veggie Bisque

Prep time: 5 minutes | Cook time: 25 minutes | Serves 6

- 1 red onion, chopped
- 2 carrots, chopped
- 1 zucchini, sliced
- 1 ripe tomato, quartered
- 2 garlic cloves, crushed
- 3 tbsp extra-virgin olive oil
- ½ tsp dried rosemary
- Sea salt and pepper to taste
- 6 cups vegetable broth
- 1 tbsp minced fresh parsley

1. Preheat your oven to 400°F. Arrange the onion, carrots, zucchini, tomato, and garlic on a greased baking dish. Sprinkle with oil, rosemary, salt, and pepper. Cover with foil and roast for 30 minutes.
2. Uncover and turn them. Roast for another 10 minutes. Transfer the veggies into a pot and pour in the broth. Bring to a boil, lower the heat and simmer for 5 minutes.
3. Transfer to a food processor and blend the soup until smooth. Return to the pot and cook until hot. Serve topped with parsley.

PER SERVING

Cal 95; Fat 7g; Carbs 8g; Protein 1g

Ginger Squash Soup

Prep time: 5 minutes | Cook time: 30 minutes | Serves 4

- 3 tsp toasted pumpkin seeds
- 1 tbsp chopped ginger paste
- 1 tbsp extra-virgin olive oil
- 1 onion, chopped
- 1 celery stalk, chopped
- 4 cups vegetable broth
- 1 acorn squash, chopped
- 1 tsp low-sodium soy sauce
- ¼ tsp ground allspice
- Sea salt and pepper to taste
- 1 cup plain soy milk

1. Heat the olive oil in a pot over medium heat. Place in onion and celery and sauté for 5 minutes until tender.
2. Add in broth and squash, bring to a boil. Lower the heat and simmer for 20 minutes. Stir in soy sauce, ginger paste, allspice, salt, and pepper.
3. Blend the soup in a food processor until smooth. Return to the pot. Mix in soy milk. Serve garnished with pumpkin seeds.

PER SERVING

Cal 195; Fat 10g; Carbs 23g; Protein 6g

Easy Garbanzo Soup

Prep time: 5 minutes | Cook time: 25 minutes | Serves 4

- 2 tbsp extra-virgin olive oil
- 1 onion, chopped
- 1 green bell pepper, diced
- 1 carrot, peeled and diced
- 4 garlic cloves, minced
- 1 (15-oz) can garbanzo beans
- 1 cup spinach, chopped
- 4 cups vegetable stock
- ¼ tsp ground cumin
- Sea salt to taste

1. Heat the oil in a pot over medium heat. Place in onion, garlic, bell pepper, and carrot and sauté for 5 minutes until tender.
2. Stir in garbanzo beans, spinach, stock, cumin, and salt. Cook for 10 minutes. Mash the garbanzo using a potato masher, leaving some chunks. Serve.

PER SERVING

Cal 120; Fat 7g; Carbs 13g; Protein 2g

Noodle Soup

Prep time: 5 minutes | Cook time: 30 minutes | Serves 6

- 4 oz soba noodles, broken into thirds
- 2 tbsp extra-virgin olive oil
- 1 onion, chopped
- 1 carrot, sliced
- 2 garlic cloves, minced
- 1 (28-oz) can diced tomatoes
- 1 cup Chana dal, rinsed
- 1 tsp dried thyme
- 6 cups vegetable broth

1. Warm the oil in a pot over medium heat. Place in onion, carrot, and garlic and sauté for 5 minutes. Add in tomatoes, chana dal, thyme, and broth.
2. Bring to a boil, then lower the heat and season with salt and pepper. Simmer for 15 minutes. Stir in soba noodles, cook 5 minutes more. Serve immediately.

PER SERVING

Cal 200; Fat 5g; Carbs 35g; Protein 5g

Hot Lentil Soup with Zucchini
Prep time: 5 minutes | Cook time: 30 minutes | Serves 4

- 2 tbsp extra-virgin olive oil
- 1 onion, chopped
- 1 zucchini, chopped
- 1 garlic clove, minced
- 1 tbsp hot paprika
- 1 (14-oz) can diced tomatoes
- 1 cup red lentils, rinsed
- 4 cups vegetable broth
- 3 cups chopped Swiss chard

1. Heat the oil in a pot over medium heat. Place in onion, zucchini, and garlic and sauté for 5 minutes until tender.
2. Add in paprika, tomatoes, lentils, broth, salt, and pepper. Bring to a boil, then lower the heat and simmer for 15 minutes, stirring often. Add in the Swiss chard and cook for another 3-5 minutes. Serve immediately.

PER SERVING

Cal 300; Fat 8g; Carbs 46g; Protein 13g

Chickpea & Vegetable Soup
Prep time: 5 minutes | Cook time: 35 minutes | Serves 5

- 2 tbsp extra-virgin olive oil
- 1 onion, chopped
- 1 carrot, chopped
- 1 celery stalk, chopped
- 1 eggplant, chopped
- 1 (28-oz) can diced tomatoes
- 2 tbsp tomato paste
- 1 (15.5-oz) can chickpeas
- 2 tsp smoked paprika
- 1 tsp ground cumin
- 1 tsp za'atar spice
- ¼ tsp cayenne pepper
- 6 cups vegetable broth
- 4 oz whole-wheat vermicelli

1. Heat oil in a pot over medium heat. Sauté the onion, carrot, and celery for 5 minutes.
2. Add the eggplant, tomatoes, tomato paste, chickpeas, paprika, cumin, za´atar spice, and cayenne pepper.
3. Stir in broth and salt. Bring to a boil and simmer for 15 minutes. Add in vermicelli and cook for another 5 minutes. Serve warm.

PER SERVING

Cal 290; Fat 8g; Carbs 50g; Protein 9g

Brussels sprouts & Tofu Soup
Prep time: 5 minutes | Cook time: 40 minutes | Serves 4

- 7 oz firm tofu, cubed
- 2 tsp olive oil
- 1 cup sliced mushrooms
- 1 lb Brussels sprouts, halved
- 1 garlic clove, minced
- ½-inch piece minced ginger
- Sea salt to taste
- 2 tbsp apple cider vinegar
- 2 tsp low-sodium soy sauce
- 1 tsp pure date sugar
- ¼ tsp red pepper flakes
- 1 scallion, chopped

1. Heat the oil in a skillet over medium heat. Place mushrooms, Brussels sprouts, garlic, ginger, and salt. Sauté for 7-8 minutes until the veggies are soft.
2. Pour in 4 cups of water, vinegar, soy sauce, sugar, pepper flakes, and tofu. Bring to a boil, then lower the heat and simmer for 5-10 minutes. Top with scallions and serve.

PER SERVING

Cal 135; Fat 8g; Carbs 8g; Protein 9g

Rosemary White Bean Soup
Prep time: 5 minutes | Cook time: 30 minutes | Serves 4

- 2 tsp olive oil
- 1 carrot, chopped
- 1 onion, chopped
- 2 garlic cloves, minced
- 1 tbsp rosemary, chopped
- 2 tbsp apple cider vinegar
- 1 cup dried white beans
- ¼ tsp sea salt
- 2 tbsp nutritional yeast

1. Heat the oil in a pot over medium heat. Place carrots, onion, and garlic and cook for 5 minutes. Pour in vinegar to deglaze the pot. Stir in 5 cups water and beans and bring to a boil.
2. Lower the heat and simmer for 45 minutes until the beans are soft. Add in salt and nutritional yeast and stir. Serve topped with chopped rosemary.

PER SERVING

Cal 225; Fat 3g; Carbs37g; Protein 14g

Coconut Mushroom Soup

Prep time: 5 minutes | Cook time: 20 minutes | Serves 2

- 2 tsp olive oil
- 1 onion, chopped
- 2 garlic cloves, minced
- 2 cups chopped mushrooms
- Sea salt and pepper to taste
- 1 tsp dried rosemary
- 4 cups vegetable broth
- 1 cup coconut cream

1. In a pot over medium heat, warm the oil. Place the onion, garlic, mushrooms, and salt and cook for 5 minutes.
2. Stir in the flour and cook for another 1-2 minutes. Add in rosemary, vegetable broth, coconut cream, and pepper. Lower the heat and simmer for 10 minutes. Serve.

PER SERVING

Cal 535; Fat 47g; Carbs 29g; Protein 10g

Rice Noodle Soup with Beans

Prep time: 5 minutes | Cook time: 10 minutes | Serves 6

- 2 carrots, chopped
- 2 celery stalks, chopped
- 6 cups vegetable broth
- 8 oz brown rice noodles
- 1 tsp dried thyme

1. Place a pot over medium heat and add in the carrots, celery, and vegetable broth. Bring to a boil.
2. Add in noodles, beans, dried thyme, salt, and pepper. Reduce the heat and simmer for 5 minutes. Serve and enjoy!

PER SERVING

Cal 210; Fat 1g; Carbs 45g; Protein 6g

Mushroom & Tofu Soup

Prep time: 5 minutes | Cook time: 20 minutes | Serves 4

- 4 cups water
- 2 tsp low-sodium soy sauce
- 4 white mushrooms, sliced
- ¼ cup minced green onions
- 3 tbsp tahini
- 6 oz extra-firm tofu, diced

1. Pour the water and soy sauce into a pot. Bring to a boil. Add in mushrooms and green onions.
2. Lower the heat and simmer for 10 minutes. In a bowl, combine ½ cup of hot soup with tahini. Pour the mixture into the pot and simmer 2 minutes, but do not boil. Stir in tofu. Serve.

PER SERVING

Cal 160; Fat 11g; Carbs 7g; Protein 7g

Pomodoro Cream Soup

Prep time: 5 minutes | Cook time: 15 minutes | Serves 5

- 1 (28-oz) can diced tomatoes
- 2 tbsp extra-virgin olive oil
- 1 tsp smoked paprika
- 2 cups vegetable broth
- 2 tsp dried herbs
- 1 red onion, chopped
- 1 cup non-dairy milk
- Sea salt and pepper to taste

1. Place the tomatoes, olive oil, paprika, broth, dried herbs, onion, milk, salt, and pepper in a pot.
2. Bring to a boil and cook for 10 minutes. Transfer to a food processor and blend the soup until smooth. Serve and enjoy!

PER SERVING

Cal 115; Fat 7g; Carbs 12g; Protein 3g

Chicken Soup with Kale

Prep time: 5 minutes | Cook time: 45 minutes | Serves 4

- 2 tbsp extra-virgin olive oil
- 1 onion, chopped
- ½ lb chicken breasts, cubed
- 4 cups vegetable broth
- 2 tbsp olive oil
- ¼ tsp cayenne pepper
- Sea salt and pepper to taste
- 4 cups kale

1. Heat the oil in a pot over medium heat. Add onion and chicken and sauté for 4-6 minutes, stirring often.
2. Pour in broth and cook for 20 minutes. Stir in cayenne pepper, salt, and pepper. Add in kale and cook 5 minutes. Serve.

PER SERVING

Cal 350; Fat 30g; Carbs 7g; Protein 13g

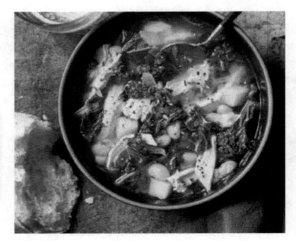

Gluten-Free Ramen "To Go"

Prep time: 10 minutes | Cook time: 5 minutes | Serves 1

- ½ cup cooked soba noodles, or soaked and drained rice noodles
- ½ cup grated carrot
- 1 large kale leaf, thoroughly washed and finely chopped
- 1 tablespoon tahini
- 1 teaspoon dried vegetable broth powder
- ⅛ teaspoon salt
- Boiling water, to cover

1. In a 1 pint mason jar, layer the soba noodles, carrot, kale, tahini, broth powder, and salt. Seal the jar. Refrigerate or pack in your lunchbox.
2. When you're ready to eat, bring a kettle of water to a boil. Fill the jar with enough water to cover the vegetables. Reseal the lid and steep the soup for 4 to 5 minutes.
3. Stir well to incorporate the seasoning, and enjoy.

PER SERVING

Calories: 206; Total Fat: 8g; Total Carbohydrates: 29g; Sugar: 3g; Fiber: 4g; Protein: 8g; Sodium: 818mg

Slow-Cooker Vegan Split Pea Soup

Prep time: 10 minutes | Cook time: 4 To 8 Hours | Serves 8

- 6½ cups water
- 2½ cups green or yellow split peas, rinsed well
- 2 small sweet potatoes, cut into ½-inch dice
- 1 tablespoon dried thyme
- 1½ teaspoons salt, plus additional as needed

1. In a slow cooker, combine the water, split peas, sweet potatoes, thyme, and salt.
2. Cover and cook on low for 8 hours, or on high for 4 hours.
3. Using an immersion blender or in a regular blender, blend half (or all) of the soup, working in batches as needed and taking care with the hot liquid.
4. Taste and adjust the seasoning, if necessary.

PER SERVING

Calories: 51; Total Fat: 0g; Total Carbohydrates: 12g; Sugar: 0g; Fiber: 2g; Protein: 1g; Sodium: 448mg

Carrot-Ginger Soup

Prep time: 5 minutes | Cook time: 35 minutes| Serves 6

- 1 large onion, peeled and roughly chopped
- 4½ cups plus 2 tablespoons water, divided
- 8 carrots, peeled and roughly chopped
- 1½-inch piece fresh ginger, sliced thin
- 1¼ teaspoons sea salt
- 2 cups unsweetened coconut milk

1. In a large pot set over medium heat, sauté the onion in 2 tablespoons of water for about 5 minutes, or until soft.
2. Add the carrots, the remaining 4½ cups of water, the ginger, and salt. Bring to a boil. Reduce the heat to low and cover the pot. Simmer for 20 minutes.
3. Stir in the coconut milk and let it heat for 4 to 5 minutes.
4. In a blender, blend the soup until creamy, working in batches if necessary and taking care with the hot liquid.

PER SERVING

Calories: 228; Total Fat: 19g; Total Carbohydrates: 15g; Sugar: 8g; Fiber: 4g; Protein: 3g; Sodium: 554mg

Cream of Broccoli Soup

Prep time: 5 minutes | Cook time: 25 minutes| Serves 6

- 1 onion, finely chopped
- 4 garlic cloves, finely chopped
- 5 cups plus 2 tablespoons water, divided
- 1½ teaspoons sea salt, plus additional as needed
- 4 broccoli heads with stalks, heads cut into florets and stalks roughly chopped
- 1 cup cashews, soaked in water for at least 4 hours

1. In a large pot set over medium heat, sauté the onion and garlic in 2 tablespoons of water for about 5 minutes, or until soft.
2. Add the remaining 5 cups of water, the salt, and the broccoli. Bring to a boil. Cover and reduce the heat to low. Simmer for 20 minutes.
3. Drain and rinse the cashews. Transfer them to a blender.
4. Add the soup to the blender. Blend until smooth, working in batches if necessary, and taking care with the hot liquid. Taste, and adjust the seasoning if necessary.

PER SERVING

Calories: 224; Total Fat: 11g; Total Carbohydrates: 26g; Sugar: 6g; Fiber: 7g; Protein: 11g; Sodium: 85mg

Classic Butternut Squash Soup

Prep time: 25 minutes | Cook time: 35 minutes| Serves 6

- 1 onion, roughly chopped
- 4½ cups plus 2 tablespoons water, divided
- 1 large butternut squash, washed, peeled, ends trimmed, halved, seeded, and cut into ½-inch chunks
- 2 celery stalks, roughly chopped
- 3 carrots, peeled and roughly chopped
- 1 teaspoon sea salt, plus additional as needed

1. In a large pot set over medium heat, sauté the onion in 2 tablespoons of water for about 5 minutes, or until soft.
2. Add the squash, celery, carrot, and salt. Bring to a boil.
3. Reduce the heat to low, Cover and simmer for 25 minutes.
4. In a blender, purée the soup until smooth, working in batches if necessary and taking care with the hot liquid. Taste, and adjust the seasoning if necessary.

PER SERVING

Calories: 104; Total Fat: 0g; Total Carbohydrates: 27g; Sugar: 6g; Fiber: 5g; Protein: 2g; Sodium: 417mg

---

Thai Sweet Potato Soup

Prep time: 10 minutes | Cook time: 20 To 25 Minutes | Serves 4

- 3 large sweet potatoes, cubed
- 2 cups water
- 1 (14-ounce) can coconut milk
- ½-inch piece fresh ginger, sliced
- ½ cup almond butter
- Zest of 1 lime
- Juice of 1 lime
- 1 teaspoon salt, plus additional as needed

1. In a large pot set over high heat, combine the sweet potatoes, water, coconut milk, and ginger. Bring to a boil. Reduce the heat to low and cover.
2. Simmer for 20 to 25 minutes, or until the potatoes are tender. Transfer the potatoes, ginger, and cooking liquid to a blender.
3. Add the almond butter, lime zest, lime juice, and salt.
4. Blend until smooth.
5. Taste, and adjust the seasoning if necessary.

PER SERVING

Calories: 653; Total Fat: 42g; Total Carbohydrates: 64g; Sugar: 4g; Fiber: 11g; Protein: 12g; Sodium: 614mg

Glorious Creamed Greens Soup

Prep time: 5 minutes | Cook time: 15 minutes| Serves 4

- 3 cups water
- 2 cups unsweetened coconut milk
- 1½ teaspoons sea salt, plus additional as needed
- 4 cups tightly packed kale, thoroughly washed, stemmed, and roughly chopped
- 4 cups tightly packed spinach, stemmed and roughly chopped
- 4 cups tightly packed collard greens, stemmed and roughly chopped
- 1 bunch fresh parsley, stemmed and roughly chopped

1. In a large pot set over high heat, bring the water, coconut milk, and salt to a boil. Reduce the heat to low.
2. Add the kale, spinach, and collard greens 1 cup at a time, letting them wilt before adding the next cup. Continue until all the greens have been added to the pot.
3. Simmer for 8 to 10 minutes.
4. In a blender, blend the soup until smooth, working in batches if necessary and taking care with the hot liquid.
5. Taste, and adjust the seasoning (if necessary) before serving.

PER SERVING

Calories: 334; Total Fat: 29g; Total Carbohydrates: 18g; Sugar: 4g; Fiber: 6g; Protein: 7g; Sodium: 959mg

---

Basic Chicken Broth (Bone Broth)

Prep time: 10 minutes | Cook time: 8 To 24 Hours | Serves 6

- 2 pounds organic chicken bones, or 1 leftover organic chicken carcass
- 1 small onion, quartered, skin on
- 1-inch piece fresh ginger, roughly chopped
- 1 small bunch fresh fennel, roughly chopped
- 1 small bunch fresh parsley, roughly chopped
- 10 to 12 cups cold water
- 1 tablespoon apple cider vinegar (optional)

1. In a slow cooker, combine the chicken bones, onion, ginger, fennel, parsley, water, and cider vinegar (if using). The amount of water needed will depend on the size of your cooker. Cover everything by 1 to 2 inches.
2. Cover and cook on low for a minimum of 8 hours.
3. Strain the broth, discarding the vegetables and bones. Cover and refrigerate until needed.

PER SERVING

Calories: 86; Total Fat: 2g; Total Carbohydrates: 8g; Sugar: 4g; Fiber: 0g; Protein: 6g; Sodium: 279mg

Comforting Chicken Stew

Prep Time: 15 minutes | Cook time: 4 Hours | Serves 4

- 1 tablespoon extra-virgin olive oil
- 3 pounds boneless, skinless chicken thighs
- 1 large onion, thinly sliced
- 2 garlic cloves, thinly sliced
- 1 teaspoon minced fresh ginger root
- 2 teaspoons ground turmeric
- 1 teaspoon whole coriander seeds, lightly crushed
- 1 teaspoon salt
- ¼ teaspoon freshly ground black pepper
- 2 cups chicken broth
- 1 cup unsweetened coconut milk
- ¼ cup chopped fresh cilantro (optional)

1. Drizzle the oil into a slow cooker.
2. Add the chicken, onion, garlic, ginger root, turmeric, coriander, salt, pepper, chicken broth, and coconut milk, and toss to combine.
3. Cover and cook on high for 4 hours. Garnish with the chopped cilantro (if using) and serve.

PER SERVING

Calories: 370; Total Fat: 19g; Total Carbohydrates: 4g; Sugar: 1g; Fiber: 1g; Protein: 46g; Sodium: 770mg

Creamy Cabbage Slaw

Prep time: 15 minutes | Cook time: 5 minutes | Serves 6

- 1 large head green or red cabbage, sliced thin
- 2 carrots, grated
- 1 cup cashews, soaked in water for at least 4 hours
- ¼ cup freshly squeezed lemon juice
- ½ to ¾ cup water
- ¾ teaspoon sea salt

1. In a large bowl, combine the cabbage and carrots.
2. Drain and rinse the cashews.
3. In a blender, process the cashews with the lemon juice, ½ cup of water, and the salt until smooth and creamy. If the dressing is too thick, add more water, 1 tablespoon at a time.
4. Pour the sauce over the vegetables and mix well. Refrigerate for at least 1 hour before serving to give the vegetables time to marinate.

PER SERVING

Calories: 208; Total Fat: 11g; Total Carbohydrates: 25g; Sugar: 4g; Fiber: 8g; Protein: 7g; Sodium: 394mg

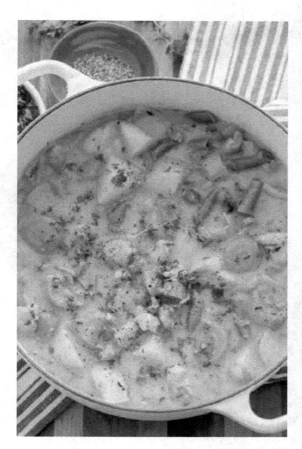

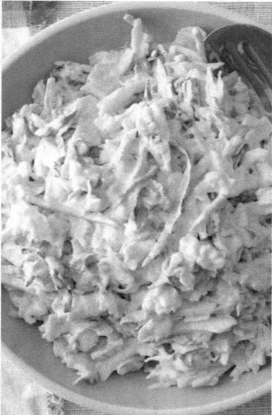

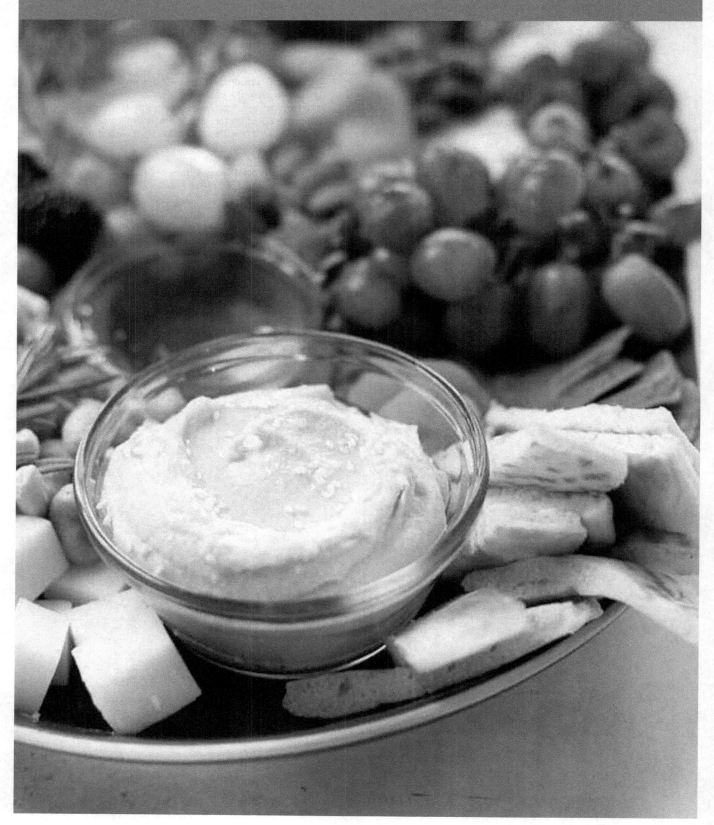

Chapter 14
Snacks & Sides

Broccoli Stir-Fry with Sesame Seeds

Prep time: 5 minutes | Cook time: 20 minutes| Serves 4

- 1 tbsp cilantro, chopped
- 2 tbsp canola oil
- 1 tsp sesame oil
- 4 cups broccoli florets
- 1 tbsp grated fresh ginger
- ¼ tsp sea salt
- 2 garlic cloves, minced
- 2 tbsp toasted sesame seeds

1. Warm the canola oil in a skillet over medium heat and place in the broccoli, ginger, garlic, and salt. Cook for 5-7 minutes until the broccoli gets brown.
2. Add in garlic and cook for another 30 seconds. Turn the heat off and mix in sesame seeds. Top with cilantro and serve immediately.

PER SERVING

Cal 140; Fat 12g; Carbs 10g; Protein 3g

Creamy Sweet Potato Slices with Chives

Prep time: 5 minutes | Cook time: 15 minutes| Serves 6

- 6 sweet potatoes, sliced
- 1 cup plain yogurt
- 2 tbsp starch
- 1 tbsp chopped chives
- 1 cup almond milk
- 1 cup chicken broth

1. Coat the sweet potatoes with salt, chives, and pepper.
2. Add broth and sweet potatoes to your Instant Pot. Seal the lid and cook on "Manual" for 5 minutes. Once the timer goes off, release the pressure quickly.
3. Carefully open the lid and transfer to a bowl. Whisk the remaining ingredients into the cooking liquid in your pot.
4. Cook for one minute, stirring constantly. Pour the sauce over the sweet potatoes. Serve and enjoy!

PER SERVING

Cal 170; Fat 3g; Carbs 30g; Protein 4g

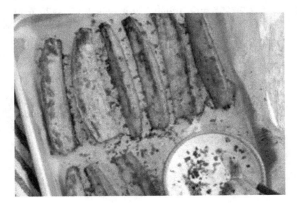

Pressure Cooked Deviled Eggs

Prep time: 5 minutes | Cook time: 20 minutes| Serves 4

- 4 eggs
- 1 tsp paprika
- 1 tbsp paleo mayonnaise
- 1 tsp Dijon mustard

1. Place the eggs and 1 cup of water in your Instant Pot. Close the lid and cook for 5 minutes on "Manual".
2. Let the pressure release naturally. Place the eggs in an ice bath and let cool for 5 minutes. Peel and cut them in half.
3. Whisk together the remaining ingredients. Top the egg halves with the mixture and enjoy!

PER SERVING

Cal 100; Fat 8g; Carbs 0.7g; Protein 6g

Spinach Chips with Guacamole Hummus

Prep time: 5 minutes | Cook time: 30 minutes | Serves 4

- ½ cup baby spinach
- 1 tbsp extra-virgin olive oil
- ½ tsp plain vinegar
- 3 large avocados, chopped
- ½ cup chopped parsley
- ½ cup extra-virgin olive oil
- ¼ cup pumpkin seeds
- ¼ cup sesame paste
- Juice from ½ lemon
- 1 garlic clove, minced
- ½ tsp coriander powder
- Sea salt and pepper to taste

1. Preheat oven to 300°F. Put spinach in a bowl and toss with olive oil, vinegar, and salt.
2. Place in a parchment paper-lined baking sheet and bake until the leaves are crispy but not burned, about 15 minutes.
3. Place avocado into the bowl of a food processor.
4. Add in parsley, olive oil, pumpkin seeds, sesame paste, lemon juice, garlic, coriander powder, salt, and black pepper. Puree until smooth. Spoon the hummus into a bowl and serve with spinach chips.

PER SERVING

Cal 655; Fat 64g; Carbs 19g; Protein 9g

Buttered Carrot Noodles with Kale
Prep time: 5 minutes | Cook time: 15 minutes| Serves 4

- 2 large carrots
- ¼ cup vegetable broth
- 4 tbsp extra-virgin olive oil
- 1 garlic clove, minced
- 1 cup chopped kale
- Sea salt and pepper to taste

1. Peel the carrots with a slicer and run both through a spiralizer to form noodles. Pour the vegetable broth into a saucepan and add the carrot noodles.
2. Simmer (over low heat) the carrots for 3 minutes. Strain through a colander and set the vegetables aside.
3. Warm the olive oil in a large skillet over medium heat. Add the garlic and sauté until softened and put in the kale; cook until wilted.
4. Pour the carrots into the pan, season with salt and black pepper, and stir-fry for 3 to 4 minutes. Serve with pan-grilled tofu.

PER SERVING

Cal 140; Fat 14g; Carbs 5g; Protein 1g

Mushroom Broccoli Faux Risotto
Prep time: 5 minutes | Cook time: 25 minutes | Serves 4

- 1 cup cremini mushrooms, chopped
- 4 oz extra-virgin olive oil
- 2 garlic cloves, minced
- 1 small red onion, chopped
- 1 large head broccoli, grated
- ¾ cup white wine
- 1 cup coconut cream
- ¾ cup grated Parmesan
- Chopped thyme

1. Warm the olive oil in a pot over medium heat. Sauté the mushrooms in the pot until golden, about 5 minutes.
2. Add the garlic and onions and cook for 3 minutes or until fragrant and soft. Mix in the broccoli, 1 cup water, and half of the white wine.
3. Season with salt and black pepper and simmer the ingredients (uncovered) for 8-10 minutes or until the broccoli is soft.
4. Mix in the coconut whipping cream and simmer until most of the cream has evaporated. Turn the heat off and stir in the parmesan cheese and thyme until well incorporated.

PER SERVING

Cal 150; Fat 9g; Carbs 12g; Protein 8g

Mixed Seed Crackers
Prep time: 5 minutes | Cook time: 60 minutes| Serves 6

- ⅓ cup sesame seed flour
- ⅓ cup pumpkin seeds
- ⅓ cup sunflower seeds
- ⅓ cup sesame seeds
- ⅓ cup chia seeds
- 1 tsp sea salt
- ¼ cup almond butter, melted

1. Preheat your oven to 300°F. Combine the sesame seed flour with pumpkin seeds, sunflower seeds, sesame seeds, chia seeds, psyllium husk powder, and salt.
2. Pour in the almond butter and 1 cup of hot water and mix the ingredients until a dough forms with a gel-like consistency.
3. Line a baking sheet with parchment paper and place the dough on the sheet. Cover the dough with another parchment paper and, with a rolling pin, flatten the dough into the baking sheet.
4. Remove the parchment paper on top. Tuck the baking sheet in the oven and bake for 45 minutes. Allow the crackers to cool and dry in the oven, about 10 minutes.
5. After, remove the sheet and break the crackers into small pieces. Serve and enjoy!

PER SERVING

Cal 470; Fat 43g; Carbs 13g; Protein 18g

Curry Cauli Rice with Mushrooms
Prep time: 5 minutes | Cook time: 15 minutes | Serves 4

- 8 oz baby Bella mushrooms, stemmed and sliced
- 1 large cauliflower head
- 2 tbsp extra-virgin olive oil
- 1 onion, chopped
- 3 garlic cloves, minced
- Sea salt and pepper to taste
- ½ tsp curry powder
- 1 tsp chopped parsley
- 2 scallions, thinly sliced

1. Use a knife to cut the entire cauliflower head into 6 pieces and transfer to a food processor. With the grater attachment, shred the cauliflower into a rice-like consistency.
2. Heat half of the olive oil in a large skillet over medium heat and then add the onion and mushrooms. Sauté for 5 minutes or until the mushrooms are soft. Add the garlic and sauté for 2 minutes or until fragrant.
3. Season with salt, black pepper, and curry powder and mix the ingredients until well combined.
4. After, turn the heat off and stir in the parsley and scallions. Serve warm.

PER SERVING

Cal 265; Fat 8g; Carbs 50g; Protein 7g

Paprika Roasted Nuts

Prep time: 5 minutes | Cook time: 10 minutes | Serves 4

- 8 oz walnuts and pecans
- 1 tsp sea salt
- 1 tbsp coconut oil
- 1 tsp cumin powder
- 1 tsp paprika powder

1. In a bowl, mix walnuts, pecans, salt, coconut oil, cumin powder, and paprika powder until the nuts are well coated with spice and oil.
2. Pour the mixture into a pan and toast while stirring continually.
3. Once the nuts are fragrant and brown, transfer to a bowl. Allow cooling and serve with chilled berry juice.

PER SERVING

Cal 400; Fat 41g; Carbs 8g; Protein 9g

Spicy Pistachio Dip

Prep time: 5 minutes | Cook time: 10 minutes| Serves 4

- 3 oz toasted pistachios,for garnish
- 3 tbsp coconut cream
- ½ lemon, juiced
- ½ tsp smoked paprika
- Cayenne pepper to taste
- ½ tsp sea salt
- ½ cup extra-virgin olive oil

1. Pour the pistachios, coconut cream, ¼ cup of water, lemon juice, paprika, cayenne pepper, and salt. Puree the ingredients at high speed until smooth.
2. Add the olive oil and puree a little further. Manage the consistency of the dip by adding more oil or water.
3. Spoon the dip into little bowls, garnish with some pistachios, and serve with julienned celery and carrots.

PER SERVING

Cal 400; Fat 40g; Carbs 8g; Protein 5g

Caramelized Pears With Yogurt

Prep Time: 15 minutes | Cook time: 10 minutes| Serves 4

- 1 tablespoon coconut oil
- 4 pears, peeled, cored, and quartered
- 2 tablespoons honey
- 1 teaspoon ground cinnamon
- ⅛ teaspoon sea salt
- 2 cups plain yogurt
- ¼ cup chopped toasted pecans (optional)

1. Heat the oil in a large skillet over medium-high heat.
2. Add the pears, honey, cinnamon, and salt, cover, and cook, stirring occasionally, until the fruit is tender, 4 to 5 minutes.
3. Uncover and let the sauce simmer for several more minutes to thicken.
4. Spoon the yogurt into four dessert bowls. Top with the warm pears, garnish with the pecans (if using), and serve.

PER SERVING

Calories: 290; Total Fat: 11g; Total Carbohydrates: 41g; Sugar: 30g; Fiber: 6g; Protein: 12g; Sodium: 110mg

Parsley Pumpkin Noodles

Prep time: 5 minutes | Cook time: 15 minutes | Serves 4

- ¼ cup extra-virgin olive oil
- ½ cup chopped onion
- 1 lb pumpkin, spiralized
- 1 bunch kale, sliced
- ¼ cup chopped parsley
- Sea salt and pepper to taste

1. Warm the olive oil in a skillet over medium heat. Place the onion and cook for 3 minutes.
2. Add in pumpkin and cook for another 7-8 minutes. Stir in kale and cook for another 2 minutes until the kale wilts.
3. Sprinkle with parsley, salt, and pepper. Serve and enjoy!

PER SERVING

Cal 780; Fat 69g; Carbs 19g; Protein 34g

Grilled Tofu Mayo Sandwiches

Prep time: 5 minutes | Cook time: 15 minutes| Serves 2

- ¼ cup paleo mayonnaise
- 2 slices whole-grain bread
- ¼ cucumber, sliced
- ½ cup lettuce, chopped
- ½ tomato, sliced
- 1 tsp extra-virgin olive oil

1. Spread the mayonnaise over a bread slice, top with the cucumber, lettuce, and tomato and finish with the other slice.
2. Heat the oil in a skillet over medium heat.
3. Place the sandwich and grill for 3 minutes, then flip over and cook for a further 3 minutes. Cut the sandwich in half.

PER SERVING

Cal 230; Fat 13g; Carbs 20g; Protein 8g

Mixed Vegetables with Basil

Prep time: 5 minutes | Cook time: 40 minutes | Serves 4

- 2/3 cup whole-wheat bread crumbs
- 2 zucchinis, chopped
- 2 yellow squashes, chopped
- 1 red onion, cut into wedges
- 1 red bell pepper, diced
- 16 cherry tomatoes, halved
- 4 tbsp extra-virgin olive oil
- Sea salt and pepper to taste
- 3 garlic cloves, minced
- 1 lemon, zested
- ¼ cup chopped basil

1. Preheat your oven to 450°F. Lightly grease a large baking sheet with cooking spray. In a medium bowl, add the zucchini, yellow squash, red onion, bell pepper, tomatoes, olive oil, salt, black pepper, and garlic.
2. Toss well and spread the mixture on the baking sheet. Roast in the oven for 25 to 30 minutes or until the vegetables are tender while stirring every 5 minutes.
3. Heat the olive oil in a medium skillet and sauté the garlic until fragrant. Mix in the breadcrumbs, lemon zest, and basil. Cook for 2 to 3 minutes. Remove the vegetables from the oven and toss in the breadcrumb's mixture.

PER SERVING

Cal 250; Fat 14g; Carbs 30g; Protein 6g

Soy Chorizo Stuffed Cabbage Rolls

Prep time: 5 minutes | Cook time: 35 minutes | Serves 4

- ¼ cup coconut oil, divided
- 1 white onion, chopped
- 3 cloves garlic, minced
- 1 cup crumbled soy chorizo
- 1 cup cauliflower rice
- 1 can tomato sauce
- 1 tsp dried oregano
- 1 tsp dried basil
- 8 green cabbage leaves

1. Heat half of the coconut oil in a saucepan over medium heat. Add half of the onion, half of the garlic, and all of the soy chorizo. Sauté for 5 minutes or until the chorizo has browned further, and the onion softened.
2. Stir in the cauli rice, season with salt and black pepper, and cook for 3 to 4 minutes. Turn the heat off.
3. Heat the remaining oil in a saucepan over medium heat, add, and sauté the remaining onion and garlic until fragrant and soft. Pour in the tomato sauce, and season with salt, black pepper, oregano, and basil.
4. Add ¼ cup water and simmer the sauce for 10 minutes. While the sauce cooks, lay the cabbage

leaves on a flat surface and spoon the soy chorizo mixture into the middle of each leaf. Roll the leaves to secure the filling.
5. Place the cabbage rolls in the tomato sauce and cook further for 10 minutes. When ready, serve the cabbage rolls with sauce over mashed broccoli or with mixed seed bread.

PER SERVING

Cal 190; Fat 15g; Carbs 10g; Protein 8g

Bell Pepper & Seitan Balls

Prep time: 5 minutes | Cook time: 25 minutes | Serves 4

- 1 egg, beaten
- 1 lb seitan, crumbled
- 1 chopped red bell peppers
- Sea salt and pepper to taste
- 1 tbsp almond flour
- 1 tsp garlic powder
- 1 tsp onion powder
- 1 tsp paleo mayonnaise
- 1 tbsp extra-virgin olive oil

1. Preheat your oven to 400°F and line a baking sheet with parchment paper.
2. In a bowl, mix the egg, seitan, bell pepper, salt, pepper, almond flour, garlic powder, onion powder, and tofu mayonnaise.
3. Mix and form 1-inch balls from the mixture.
4. Arrange on the baking sheet, brush with cooking spray, and bake in the oven for 15-20 minutes or until brown and compacted. Serve warm.

PER SERVING

Cal 490; Fat 40g; Carbs 4g; Protein 29g

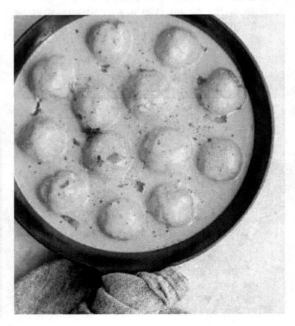

Tomatoes Stuffed with Chickpeas & Quinoa

Prep time: 5 minutes | Cook time: 50 minutes | Serves 4

- 8 medium tomatoes
- ¾ cup quinoa
- 1½ cups water
- 1 tbsp extra-virgin olive oil
- 1 small onion, diced
- 3 garlic cloves, minced
- 1 cup chopped spinach
- 1 (7 oz) can chickpeas
- ½ cup chopped basil

1. Preheat your oven to 400°F. Cut off the heads of tomatoes and use a paring knife to scoop the inner pulp of the tomatoes. Season with some olive oil, salt, and black pepper.
2. Add the quinoa and water to a medium pot, season with salt, and cook until the quinoa is tender and the water absorbs, 10-15 minutes. Fluff and set aside.
3. Heat the remaining olive oil in a skillet and sauté the onion and garlic for 30 seconds.
4. Mix in the spinach and cook until wilted, 2 minutes. Stir in the basil, chickpeas, and quinoa; allow warming from 2 minutes.
5. Spoon the mixture into the tomatoes, place the tomatoes into the baking dish and bake in the oven for 20 minutes or until the tomatoes soften. Serve and enjoy!

PER SERVING

Cal 290; Fat 8g; Carbs 47g; Protein 12g

Divine Roasted Chickpeas

Prep time: 5 minutes | Cook time: 1 hour 35 minutes | Serves 6

- 1 tsp curry powder
- 2 tsp extra-virgin olive oil
- 1 cup chickpeas, soaked
- 1 tbsp garlic powder
- 1 tsp onion powder
- ¾ tsp sea salt

1. Put the chickpeas in a large pot over medium heat and cover with a few inches of water. Bring to a boil. Cook for about 45 minutes until tender. Drain again.
2. Preheat your oven to 325°F. Line a large baking sheet with aluminum foil.
3. In a large bowl, toss together the chickpeas, curry powder, olive oil, garlic powder, onion powder, and salt. Taste and adjust the seasoning if necessary. Remember that the flavors intensify as the chickpeas bake.
4. Spread the chickpeas onto the prepared sheet. Depending on the size of your sheet, you may need two.
5. Carefully place the sheet (s) in the preheated oven and bake for about 45 minutes, stirring and turning the chickpeas every 15 minutes, or until golden and crunchy. The chickpeas will also crisp as they cool.

PER SERVING

Cal 105; Fat 3g; Carbs 15g; Protein 5g

Mustard Tofu Avocado Wraps

Prep time: 5 minutes | Cook time: 25 minutes | Serves 4

- 3 cups shredded romaine lettuce
- 6 tbsp extra-virgin olive oil
- 1 lb tofu, cut into strips
- 1 tsp low-sodium soy sauce
- ¼ cup apple cider vinegar
- 1 tsp yellow mustard
- 3 ripe Roma tomatoes, diced
- 1 large carrot, shredded
- 1 avocado, chopped
- 1 minced red onion
- ¼ cup sliced green olives
- 4 whole-grain flour tortillas

1. Heat 2 tbsp of olive oil in a skillet over medium heat. Place the tofu, cook for 10 minutes until golden brown.
2. Drizzle with soy sauce. Let cool. In a bowl, whisk the vinegar, mustard, salt, pepper, and the remaining oil. In another bowl, mix the lettuce, tomatoes, carrot, avocado, onion, and olives.
3. Pour the dressing over the salad and toss to coat.
4. Lay out a tortilla on a clean flat surface and spoon ¼ of the salad, some tofu, and then roll up. Cut in half. Repeat the process with the remaining tortillas.

PER SERVING

Cal 405; Fat 35g; Carbs 16g; Protein 14g

Dijon Roasted Asparagus

Prep time: 5 minutes | Cook time: 35 minutes | Serves 4

- 2 tbsp extra-virgin olive oil
- 1 lb asparagus, trimmed
- 2 garlic cloves, minced
- 1 tsp Dijon mustard
- 1 tbsp lemon juice

1. Warm the olive oil in a large skillet and sauté the asparagus until softened with some crunch, 7 minutes.
2. Mix in the garlic and cook until fragrant, 30 seconds.
3. In a small bowl, quickly whisk the mustard, lemon juice and pour the mixture over the asparagus. Cook for 2 minutes. Plate the asparagus. Serve warm.

PER SERVING

Cal 90; Fat 7g; Carbs 5g; Protein 3g

Vegetable & Rice Vermicelli Lettuce Rolls

Prep time: 5 minutes | Cook time: 15 minutes | Serves 4

- ½ cucumber, sliced lengthwise
- ½ red bell pepper, cut into strips
- 2 green onions, sliced
- 2 tbsp extra-virgin olive oil
- 2 tsp low-sodium soy sauce
- 2 tbsp balsamic vinegar
- 1 tsp pure date sugar
- ⅛ tsp crushed red pepper
- 3 oz rice vermicelli
- 6 green leaf lettuce leaves
- 1 medium carrot, shredded
- 1 cup cilantro leaves

1. Separate the white part of the green onions, chop and transfer to a bowl.
2. Stir in soy sauce, balsamic vinegar, date sugar, red pepper, and 3 tbsp water. Set aside. Submerge the vermicelli in a bowl with hot water for 4 minutes.
3. Drain and mix with olive oil. Allow cooling. Put the lettuce leaves on a flat surface.
4. Divide rice noodles between the lettuce leaves and top with green onions, carrot, cucumber, bell pepper, and cilantro. Roll the leaves up from the smaller edges. Serve with dipping sauce.

PER SERVING

Cal 155; Fat 7g; Carbs 22g; Protein 1g

Paprika Tofu & Zucchini Skewers

Prep time: 5 minutes | Cook time: 10 minutes | Serves 4

- 1 (14 oz) block tofu, cubed
- 1 zucchini, cut into rounds
- 1 tbsp extra-virgin olive oil
- 2 tbsp lemon juice
- 1 tsp smoked paprika
- 1 tsp cumin powder
- 1 tsp garlic powder
- Sea salt and pepper to taste

1. Preheat a grill to medium heat. Meanwhile, thread the tofu and zucchini alternately on the wooden skewers.
2. In a small bowl, whisk the olive oil, lemon juice, paprika, cumin powder, and garlic powder. Brush the skewers all around with the mixture and place on the grill grate.
3. Cook on both sides until golden brown, 5 minutes. Season with salt and pepper and serve afterward.

PER SERVING

Cal 115; Fat 8g; Carbs 5g; Protein 8g

Chocolate Bars with Walnuts

Prep time: 5 minutes | Cook time: 60 minutes | Serves 4

- 1 cup walnuts
- 3 tbsp sunflower seeds
- 2 tbsp dark chocolate chips
- 1 tbsp cocoa powder
- 1 ½ tsp vanilla extract
- ¼ tsp cinnamon powder
- 2 tbsp melted coconut oil
- 2 tbsp toasted almond meal
- 2 tsp pure maple syrup

1. In a food processor, add the walnuts, sunflower seeds, chocolate chips, cocoa powder, vanilla extract, cinnamon powder, coconut oil, almond meal, maple syrup, and blitz a few times until combined.
2. Line a flat baking sheet with plastic wrap, pour the mixture onto the sheet and place another plastic wrap on top.
3. Use a rolling pin to flatten the batter and then remove the top plastic wrap.
4. Freeze the snack until firm, 1 hour. Remove from the freezer, cut into 1 ½-inch sized bars and enjoy immediately.

PER SERVING

Cal 300; Fat 26g; Carbs 20g; Protein 5g

Kale Chips

Prep Time: 15 minutes | Cook time: 20 minutes | Serves 4

- 1 large bunch kale, washed and thoroughly dried, stems removed, leaves cut into 2-inch pieces
- 2 tablespoons extra-virgin olive oil
- 1 teaspoon sea salt

1. Preheat the oven to 275°F.
2. In a large bowl, use your hands to mix the kale and olive oil until the kale is evenly coated.
3. Transfer the kale to a large baking sheet and sprinkle the sea salt over it.
4. Bake, turning the kale leaves once halfway through, until crispy, about 20 minutes.

PER SERVING

Calories: 88; Total Fat: 7.2g; Total Carbohydrates: 5.7g; Sugar: 1.3g; Fiber: 2g; Protein: 1.9g; Sodium: 605mg

Chickpea Paste

Prep Time: 15 Minutes, Plus 30 Minutes To Sit | Makes about 2 cups

- 1 (15-ounce) can chickpeas, drained and rinsed
- ¼ cup extra-virgin olive oil
- ¼ cup fresh lemon juice
- ¼ cup minced onion
- 1 garlic clove, minced
- 1 teaspoon sea salt
- ½ teaspoon ground cumin
- ¼ teaspoon red pepper flakes

1. In a medium bowl, use a potato masher to mash the chickpeas until they are mostly broken up.
2. Add the olive oil, lemon juice, onion, garlic, salt, cumin, and red pepper flakes and continue mashing until you have a slightly chunky paste. Let sit for 30 minutes at room temperature for the flavors to develop, then serve.

PER SERVING

Calories: 110; Total Fat: 8g; Total Carbohydrates: 10g; Sugar: 2g; Fiber: 2g; Protein: 3g; Sodium: 290mg

Spiced Nuts

Prep time: 10 minutes | Cook time: 15 minutes | Makes about 2 cups

- 1 cup almonds
- ½ cup walnuts
- ¼ cup sunflower seeds
- ¼ cup pumpkin seeds
- 1 teaspoon ground turmeric
- ½ teaspoon ground cumin
- ¼ teaspoon garlic powder
- ¼ teaspoon red pepper flakes

1. Preheat the oven to 350°F.
2. Combine all the ingredients in a medium bowl and mix well.
3. Spread the nuts evenly on a rimmed baking sheet and bake until lightly toasted, 10 to 15 minutes.
4. Cool completely before serving or storing.

PER SERVING

Calories: 180; Total Fat: 16g; Total Carbohydrates: 7g; Sugar: 1g; Fiber: 3g; Protein: 6g; Sodium: <5mg

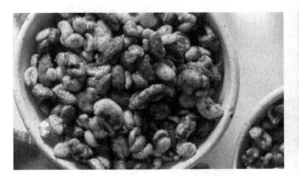

Coconut-Mango Lassi

Prep Time: 10 minutes | Serves 2

- 1½ cups frozen mango chunks
- 1 cup unsweetened coconut milk
- 1 cup ice cubes
- ½ cup plain yogurt
- 1 tablespoon honey
- Pinch ground cardamom

1. Combine the mango, coconut milk, ice cubes, yogurt, and honey in a blender and blend until smooth.
2. Pour into two tall glasses. Sprinkle a little ground cardamom over each drink and serve.

PER SERVING

Calories: 370; Total Fat: 26g; Total Carbohydrates: 32g; Sugar: 27g; Fiber: 2g; Protein: 8g; Sodium: 30mg

Avocado Fudge

Prep Time: 15 Minutes, Plus 3 Hours To Chill | Makes 16 Pieces

- 1½ cup bittersweet chocolate chips
- ¼ cup coconut oil
- 1 ripe avocado, peeled and pitted
- ½ teaspoon sea salt

1. Line an 8-inch square baking pan with waxed or parchment paper.
2. In a double boiler (not the microwave), melt the chocolate and coconut oil.
3. Once melted, transfer to the bowl of a food processor and let them cool a bit. (If the chocolate is too hot when combined with the avocado, the mixture will separate.) Add the avocado and process until smooth.
4. Spoon the mixture into the lined pan, sprinkle with the sea salt, and chill for 3 hours. Cut into 16 pieces and serve.

PER SERVING

Calories: 120; Total Fat: 9g; Total Carbohydrates: 11g; Sugar: 9g; Fiber: 2g; Protein: 1g; Sodium: 80mg

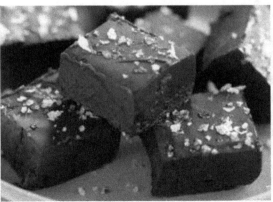

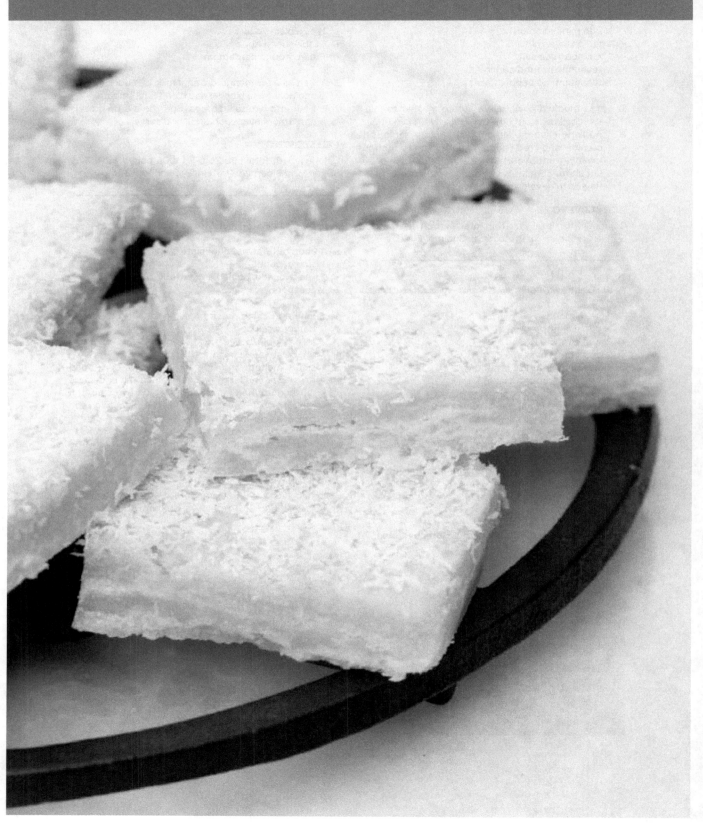

Melon with Berry-Yogurt Sauce

Prep time: 5 minutes | Cook time: 15 minutes | Serves 6

- 1 cantaloupe, peeled and sliced
- 1 pint fresh raspberries
- ½ teaspoon vanilla extract
- 1 cup plain coconut or almond yogurt
- ½ cup toasted coconut

1. Arrange the melon slices on a serving plate.
2. In a small bowl, mash the berries with the vanilla. Add the yogurt and stir until just mixed.
3. Spoon the berry-yogurt mixture over the melon slices and sprinkle with the coconut.

PER SERVING

Calories: 76; Total Fat: 4g;Total Carbohydrates: 11g;Sugar: 5g; Fiber: 6g;Protein: 1g; Sodium: 37mg

Roasted Peaches with Raspberry Sauce and Coconut Cream

Prep time: 5 minutes | Cook time: 15 minutes | Serves 4

- 4 peaches, almost ripe, halved
- 2 tablespoons coconut oil, melted
- 1 (10-ounce) bag frozen no-added-sugar raspberries, thawed
- ½ cup coconut cream
- 2 tablespoons chopped pistachios

1. Preheat the oven to 400°F.
2. In a shallow baking dish, place the peaches and brush them with the melted coconut oil.
3. Place the dish in the preheated oven and roast the peaches for 10 to 15 minutes, or until they begin to brown.
4. While the peaches are roasting, purée the raspberries in a food processor. If you don't like seeds in your raspberry sauce, strain it through a fine-mesh strainer.
5. To serve, place the peaches on a serving platter, cut-side up. Top with Coconut Cream, drizzle with raspberry sauce, and sprinkle with the pistachios.

PER SERVING

Calories: 261; Total Fat: 16g;Total Carbohydrates: 31g;Sugar: 25g; Fiber: 6g;Protein: 3g; Sodium: 5mg

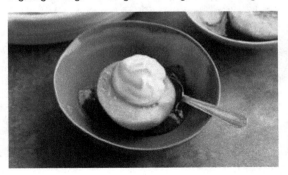

Cherry Ice Cream

Prep time: 5 minutes | Cook time: 15 minutes | Serves 4

- 1 (10-ounce) package frozen no-added-sugar cherries
- 3 cups unsweetened almond milk
- 1 teaspoon vanilla extract
- ½ teaspoon almond extract

1. In a blender or food processor, combine the cherries, almond milk, vanilla extract, and almond extract. Process until mostly smooth; a few chunks of cherries are fine.
2. Pour the mixture into a container with an airtight lid. Freeze thoroughly before serving.

PER SERVING

Calories: 82; Total Fat: 2g;Total Carbohydrates: 14g;-Sugar: 12g; Fiber: 2g;Protein: 1g; Sodium: 121mg

Blueberry Crisp

Prep time: 5 minutes | Cook time: 25 minutes | Serves 4

- ½ cup coconut oil, melted, plus additional for brushing
- 1 quart fresh blueberries
- ¼ cup maple syrup
- Juice of ½ lemon
- 2 teaspoons lemon zest
- 1 cup gluten-free rolled oats
- ½ teaspoon ground cinnamon
- ½ cup chopped pecans
- Pinch salt

1. Preheat the oven to 350°F.
2. Brush a shallow baking dish with melted coconut oil. Stir together the blueberries, maple syrup, lemon juice, and lemon zest in the dish.
3. In a small bowl, combine the oats, ½ cup of melted coconut oil, cinnamon, pecans, and salt. Mix the ingredients well to evenly distribute the coconut oil. Sprinkle the oat mixture over the berries.
4. Place the dish in the preheated oven and bake for 20 minutes, or until the oats are lightly browned.

PER SERVING

Calories: 497; Total Fat: 33g;Total Carbohydrates: 51g;Sugar: 26g; Fiber: 7g;Protein: 5g; Sodium: 42mg

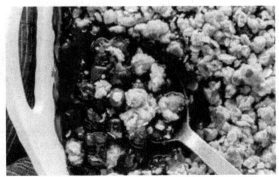

Grilled Pineapple with Chocolate Ganache

Prep time: 15 minutes | Cook time: 15 minutes| Serves 4

FOR THE GANACHE

- ½ cup coconut milk
- 1½ cups semi-sweet or bittersweet chocolate morsels
- FOR THE PINEAPPLE
- 1 pineapple, peeled, cored, and cut into 16 wedges
- 1 tablespoon coconut oil, melted
- 1 tablespoon coconut sugar
- 1 teaspoon chopped fresh rosemary

TO MAKE THE GANACHE

1. In a medium saucepan over medium-high heat, add the coconut milk. Heat the milk until it just begins to scald (little bubbles or foam will begin to collect around the perimeter of the pan).
2. Remove the pan from the heat and add the chocolate. Let stand for 1 minute.
3. Whisk the mixture until it's smooth and satiny.

TO MAKE THE PINEAPPLE

1. Preheat an indoor stove-top grill until very hot.
2. Brush the pineapple wedges with melted coconut oil.
3. Grill the wedges for 1 to 2 minutes per side, or until grill marks appear.
4. Arrange the pineapple on a serving platter and sprinkle with the coconut sugar and rosemary.
5. Serve with the ganache.

PER SERVING

Calories: 462; Total Fat: 23g;Total Carbohydrates: 61g;Sugar: 48g; Fiber: 2g;Protein: 5g; Sodium: 5mg

Chocolate-Avocado Mousse with Sea Salt

Prep time: 5 minutes | Cook time: 15 minutes| Serves 4

- 8 ounces bittersweet chocolate, chopped
- ¼ cup coconut milk
- 2 tablespoons coconut oil
- 2 ripe avocados
- ¼ cup raw honey or maple syrup
- Pinch sea salt

1. In a small heavy saucepan over low heat, combine the chocolate, coconut milk, and coconut oil. Cook for 2 to 3 minutes, stirring constantly, or until the chocolate melts.
2. In a food processor, combine the avocado and honey. Add the melted chocolate and process until smooth.
3. Spoon the mousse into serving bowls and top each with a sprinkle of sea salt. Chill for at least 30 minutes before serving.

PER SERVING

Calories: 653; Total Fat: 47g;Total Carbohydrates: 56g;Sugar: 42g; Fiber: 9g;Protein: 7g; Sodium: 113mg

Fruit and Walnut Crumble

Prep time: 15 minutes | Cook time: 15 minutes| Serves 6

FOR THE TOPPING

- 1 cup coarsely chopped walnuts
- ¼ cup coarsely chopped hazelnuts
- 1 tablespoon ghee or melted coconut oil
- 1 teaspoon ground cinnamon
- Pinch salt

FOR THE FILLING

- 1 cup fresh blueberries
- 6 fresh figs, quartered
- 2 nectarines, pitted and sliced
- ½ cup coconut sugar, raw honey, or maple syrup
- 2 teaspoons lemon zest
- 1 teaspoon vanilla extract

TO MAKE THE TOPPING

1. In a small bowl, mix together the walnuts, hazelnuts, ghee, cinnamon, and salt. Set aside.

TO MAKE THE FILLING

1. Preheat the oven to 375°F.
2. In a medium bowl, combine the blueberries, figs, nectarines, coconut sugar, lemon zest, and vanilla.
3. Divide the fruit among six ovenproof single-serving bowls or ramekins.
4. Spoon equal amounts of the nut topping over each serving.
5. Place the bowls in the preheated oven and bake for 15 to 20 minutes, or until the nuts brown and the fruit is bubbly.

PER SERVING

Calories: 335; Total Fat: 19g;Total Carbohydrates: 42g;Sugar: 32g; Fiber: 6g;Protein: 6g; Sodium: 32mg

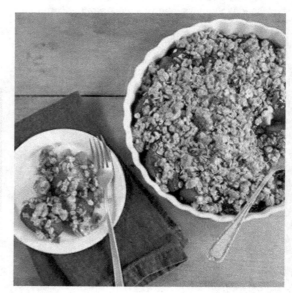

Coconut Ice Cream Sandwiches

Prep time: 45 minutes | Cook time: 15 minutes| Serves 4

FOR THE COCONUT

- ICE CREAM
- 4 cups full-fat coconut milk
- ¾ cup coconut sugar
- 2 teaspoons vanilla extract

FOR THE COOKIES

- 2 cups almond flour
- 3 tablespoons coconut sugar
- 6 tablespoons coconut oil, melted and cooled slightly
- ¼ cup maple syrup
- 1 tablespoon almond milk
- 1 teaspoon vanilla extract

FOR THE FINISHED

- ICE CREAM SANDWICHES
- ½ cup shredded coconut

TO MAKE THE COCONUT ICE CREAM

1. In a large saucepan over medium heat, combine the coconut milk and coconut sugar. Cook for about 5 minutes, stirring constantly, or until the sugar dissolves. Remove the pan from the heat and stir in the vanilla.
2. Chill the mixture for at least 4 hours, or overnight.
3. Make the ice cream according to the manufacturer's instructions for your ice cream maker.
4. Freeze the ice cream in an airtight container.

TO MAKE THE COOKIES

1. Preheat the oven to 325°F.
2. Line two baking sheets with parchment paper.
3. In a medium bowl, combine the almond flour, coconut sugar, salt, baking soda, and cardamom.
4. Add the coconut oil, maple syrup, almond milk, and vanilla. Mix until a thick dough forms.
5. Using a spoon, place scoops of dough on the prepared sheets, leaving about 2 inches between each cookie. There should be enough dough for 12 cookies.
6. Gently flatten the cookies with your hand or the back of the spoon.
7. Place the sheets in the preheated oven and bake for 10 to 12 minutes, or until golden brown. Cool the cookies thoroughly before making the ice cream sandwiches.

TO ASSEMBLE THE ICE CREAM SANDWICHES

1. Place a generous scoop of coconut ice cream on the bottom of one cookie and top it with a second cookie, pressing together gently. Individually wrap the cookies and freeze until ready to eat.
2. When ready to serve, press shredded coconut into the ice cream along the edges of each sandwich.

PER SERVING

Calories: 673; Total Fat: 53g;Total Carbohydrates: 48g;- Sugar: 42g; Fiber: 2g;Protein: 5g; Sodium: 538mg

Chocolate-Cherry Clusters

Prep time: 15 minutes | Cook time: 15 minutes|Makes about 10 clusters

- 1 cup dark chocolate (60 percent cocoa or higher), chopped
- 1 tablespoon coconut oil
- 1 cup roasted salted almonds
- ½ cup dried cherries

1. Line a rimmed baking sheet with wax paper.
2. Over a double boiler, stir together the chocolate and coconut oil until melted and smooth.
3. Remove the pan from the heat and stir in the almonds and cherries.
4. By spoonfuls, drop clusters onto the wax paper. Refrigerate until hardened.
5. Transfer to an airtight container and refrigerate.

PER SERVING

Calories: 198; Total Fat: 13g;Total Carbohydrates: 18g;Sugar: 12g; Fiber: 4g;Protein: 4g; Sodium: 58mg

Gluten-Free Oat and Fruit Bars

Prep time: 15 minutes | Cook time: 45 minutes|Makes 16 bars

- Cooking spray
- ½ cup maple syrup
- ½ cup almond or sunflower butter
- 2 medium ripe bananas, mashed
- ⅓ cup dried cranberries
- 1½ cups old-fashioned rolled oats
- ½ cup shredded coconut
- ¼ cup oat flour
- ¼ cup ground flaxseed
- 1 teaspoon vanilla extract
- ½ teaspoon ground cinnamon
- ¼ teaspoon ground cloves

1. Preheat the oven to 400°F.
2. Line an 8-by-8-inch square pan with parchment paper or aluminum foil, and coat the lined pan with cooking spray.
3. In a medium bowl, combine the maple syrup, almond butter, and bananas. Mix until well blended.
4. Add the cranberries, oats, coconut, oat flour, flaxseed, vanilla, cinnamon, and cloves. Mix well.
5. Spoon the mixture into the prepared pan; the mixture will be thick and sticky. Use an oiled spatula to spread the mixture evenly.
6. Place the pan in the preheated oven and bake for 40 to 45 minutes, or until the top is dry and a toothpick inserted in the middle comes out clean. Cool completely before cutting into bars.

PER SERVING

Calories: 144; Total Fat: 7g;Total Carbohydrates: 19g;Sugar: 8g; Fiber: 2g;Protein: 3g; Sodium: 3mg

Milk Dumplings in Cardamom Sauce

Prep time: 5 minutes | Cook time: 30 minutes | Serves 6

- 2 ½ cups brown sugar
- 3 tbsp lime juice
- 6 cups almond milk
- 1 tsp ground cardamom

1. Place the milk in a pot inside your Instant Pot and bring it to a boil. Stir in the lime juice. The solids should start to separate.
2. Pour the milk through a cheesecloth-lined colander. Drain as much liquid as you possibly can.
3. Place the paneer on a smooth surface. Form a ball and then divide it into 20 equal pieces.
4. Pour 6 cups of water into your pressure cooker and bring it to a boil. Add the sugar and cardamom and cook until dissolved. Shape the dumplings into balls, and place them in the syrup.
5. Close the lid and cook on "Manual" for about 4-5 minutes. Let cool and then refrigerate until ready to serve.

PER SERVING

Cal 135; Fat 1.5g; Carbs 12g; Protein 2g

Aunt's Apricot Tarte Tatin

Prep time: 5 minutes | Cook time: 30 minutes + cooling time | Serves 4

- 4 eggs
- ¼ cup almond flour
- 3 tbsp whole-wheat flour
- ½ tsp sea salt
- ¼ cup cold almond butter, crumbled
- 3 tbsp pure maple syrup
- 4 tbsp melted almond butter
- 3 tsp pure maple syrup
- 1 tsp vanilla extract
- 1 lemon, juiced
- 12 pitted apricots, halved
- ½ cup coconut cream
- 4 fresh basil leaves

1. Preheat your oven to 350°F. Grease a large pie pan with cooking spray. In a large bowl, combine the flours and salt. Add the melted almond butter, and using an electric hand mixer, whisk until crumbly.
2. Pour in the eggs and maple syrup and mix until smooth dough forms. Flatten the dough on a flat surface, cover with plastic wrap, and refrigerate for 1 hour. Dust a working surface with almond flour, remove the dough onto the surface, and using a rolling pin, flatten the dough into a 1-inch diameter circle. Set aside.
3. In a large bowl, mix the almond butter, maple syrup, vanilla, and lemon juice. Add the apricots to the mixture and coat well.
4. Arrange the apricots (open side down) in the pie pan and lay the dough on top. Press to fit and cut

off the dough hanging on the edges. Bake in the oven for 35 to 40 minutes or until golden brown and puffed up.
5. Remove the pie pan from the oven, allow cooling for 5 minutes, and run a butter knife around the edges of the pastry.
6. Invert the dessert onto a large plate, spread the coconut cream on top, and garnish with basil leaves. Serve sliced.

PER SERVING

Cal 535; Fat 38g; Carbs 49g; Protein 5g

Vanilla Berry Tarts

Prep time: 5 minutes | Cook time: 35 minutes + cooling time | Serves 4

- 4 eggs, beaten
- 1/3 cup whole-wheat flour
- ½ tsp salt
- ¼ cup almond butter
- 3 tbsp pure malt syrup
- 6 oz coconut cream
- 6 tbsp pure date sugar
- ¾ tsp vanilla extract
- 1 cup mixed frozen berries

1. Preheat your oven to 350°F. In a large bowl, combine flour and salt. Add almond butter and whisk until crumbly.
2. Pour in the eggs and malt syrup and mix until smooth dough forms. Flatten the dough on a flat surface, cover with plastic wrap, and refrigerate for 1 hour.
3. Dust a working surface with some flour, remove the dough onto the surface, and using a rolling pin, flatten the dough into a 1-inch diameter circle.
4. Use a large cookie cutter, cut out rounds of the dough and fit into the pie pans.
5. Use a knife to trim the edges of the pan. Lay a parchment paper on the dough cups, pour on some baking beans, and bake in the oven until golden brown, 15-20 minutes.
6. Remove the pans from the oven, pour out the baking beans, and allow cooling. In a bowl, mix coconut cream, date sugar, and vanilla extract.
7. Divide the mixture into the tart cups and top with berries. Serve.

PER SERVING

Cal 590; Fat 38g; Carbs 56g; Protein 13g

Vanilla Brownies

Prep time: 5 minutes | Cook time: 30 minutes + chilling time| Serves 4

- 2 eggs
- ¼ cup cocoa powder
- ½ cup almond flour
- ½ tsp baking powder
- ½ cup stevia
- 10 tbsp almond butter
- 2 oz dark chocolate
- ½ tsp vanilla extract

1. Preheat your oven to 375°F. In a bowl, mix cocoa powder, almond flour, baking powder, and stevia until no lumps.
2. In another bowl, add the almond butter and dark chocolate and melt both in the microwave for 30 seconds to 1 minute.
3. Whisk the eggs and vanilla into the chocolate mixture, then pour the mixture into the dry ingredients. Combine evenly.
4. Pour the batter onto a paper-lined baking sheet and bake for 20 minutes. Cool completely and refrigerate for 2 hours. When ready, slice into squares and serve.

PER SERVING

Cal 300; Fat 32g; Carbs 6g; Protein 3g

Lime Avocado Ice Cream

Prep time: 5 minutes | Cook time: 10 minutes| Serves 4

- 2 large avocados, pitted
- Juice and zest of 3 limes
- 1/3 cup stevia
- 1 ¾ cups coconut cream
- ¼ tsp vanilla extract

1. In a blender, combine the avocado pulp, lime juice and zest, stevia, coconut cream, and vanilla extract. Process until the mixture is smooth.
2. Pour the mixture into your ice cream maker and freeze based on the manufacturer's instructions.
3. When ready, remove and scoop the ice cream into bowls. Serve immediately.

PER SERVING

Cal 515; Fat 51g; Carbs 18g; Protein 6g

Crème Caramel Coconut Flan

Prep time: 5 minutes | Cook time: 30 minutes| Serves 4

- 2 eggs
- 7 oz coconut milk
- ½ cups coconut milk
- ½ tsp vanilla
- 1 cup brown sugar

1. Place a pan with a heavy bottom in your Instant Pot. Place the sugar in the pan. Cook until a caramel is formed. Divide the caramel between 4 small ramekins.
2. Pour 1 cup of water into the pressure cooker and lower the trivet. Beat the rest of the ingredients together and divide them between the ramekins.
3. Cover them with aluminum foil and place in the pot. Close the lid and cook for 5 minutes on "Manual".
4. Release the pressure naturally for 10 minutes. Serve and enjoy!

PER SERVING

Cal 110; Fat 3g; Carbs 16g; Protein 3g

Raspberries Turmeric Panna Cotta

Prep time: 5 minutes | Cook time:10 minutes + chilling time| Serves 6

- ½ tbsp powdered gelatin
- 2 cups coconut cream
- ¼ tsp vanilla extract
- 1 pinch turmeric powder
- 1 tbsp stevia
- 1 tbsp minced toasted pecans
- 12 fresh raspberries

1. Mix gelatin and ½ tsp water and allow sitting to dissolve.
2. Pour coconut cream, vanilla extract, turmeric, and stevia into a saucepan and bring to a boil over medium heat, then simmer for 2 minutes.
3. Turn the heat off. Stir in the gelatin until dissolved. Pour the mixture into 6 glasses, cover with plastic wrap, and refrigerate for 2 hours or more.
4. Top with the pecans and raspberries and serve.

PER SERVING

Cal 275; Fat 29g; Carbs 6g; Protein 3g

Summer Banana Pudding

Prep time: 5 minutes | Cook time: 25 minutes + cooling time| Serves 4

- 1 cup almond milk
- 2 cups coconut cream
- ¾ cup date sugar
- ¼ tsp salt
- 3 tbsp arrowroot
- 2 tbsp almond butter
- 1 tsp vanilla extract
- 2 bananas, sliced

1. In a medium pot, mix almond milk, coconut cream, date sugar, and salt. Cook over medium heat until slightly thickened, 10-15 minutes.
2. Stir in the arrowroot, almond butter, vanilla extract, and banana extract.
3. Cook further for 1-2 minutes or until the pudding thickens.
4. Dish the pudding into 4 serving bowls and chill in the refrigerator for at least 1 hour. To serve, top with the bananas.

PER SERVING

Cal 410; Fat 43g; Carbs 9g; Protein 5g

Avocado Truffles with Chocolate Coating

Prep time: 5 minutes | Cook time: 5 minutes| Serves 6

- 1 ripe avocado, pitted
- ½ tsp vanilla extract
- ½ tsp lemon zest
- 5 oz dark chocolate
- 1 tbsp coconut oil
- 1 tbsp cocoa powder

1. Scoop the pulp of the avocado into a bowl and mix with the vanilla using an immersion blender.
2. Stir in the lemon zest and a pinch of salt.
3. Pour the chocolate and coconut oil into a safe microwave bowl and melt in the microwave for 1 minute. Add to the avocado mixture and stir.
4. Allow cooling to firm up a bit. Form balls out of the mix. Roll each ball in the cocoa powder and serve immediately.

PER SERVING

Cal 85; Fat 7g; Carbs 5g; Protein 1g

Chocolate & Peanut Butter Cookies

Prep time: 5 minutes | Cook time: 15 minutes + cooling time| Serves 4

- 1 egg, beaten
- 1 cup pure date sugar
- 1 cup peanut butter, softened
- 1 tsp vanilla extract
- 1 ¾ cup whole-wheat flour
- 1 tsp baking soda
- ¼ tsp salt
- ¼ cup dark chocolate chips

1. In a medium bowl, whisk ½ cup of date sugar, peanut butter until light and fluffy. Mix in the egg and vanilla until combined.
2. Add in flour, baking soda, salt, and whisk well again. Fold in chocolate chips, cover the bowl with plastic wrap, and refrigerate for 1 hour.
3. Preheat oven to 375°F and line a baking sheet with parchment paper. Use a cookie sheet to scoop mounds of the batter onto the sheet with 1-inch intervals.
4. Bake for 10 minutes. Remove the cookies from the oven, cool for 3 minutes, roll in the remaining date sugar, and serve.

PER SERVING

Cal 690; Fat 43g; Carbs 69g; Protein 16g

Coconut & Chocolate Cake

Prep time: 5 minutes | Cook time: 40 minutes + cooling time| Serves 4

- 2/3 cup almond flour
- ¼ cup almond butter, melted
- 2 cups chocolate bars, cubed
- 2 ½ cups coconut cream
- Fresh berries for topping

1. Mix the almond flour and almond butter in a medium bowl and pour the mixture into a greased springform pan.
2. Use the spoon to spread and press the mixture into the pan. Place in the refrigerator to firm for 30 minutes.
3. Meanwhile, pour the chocolate in a safe microwave bowl and melt for 1 minute stirring every 30 seconds. Remove from the microwave and mix in the coconut cream and maple syrup.
4. Remove the cake pan from the oven, pour the chocolate mixture on top, and shake the pan and even the layer. Chill further for 4 to 6 hours.
5. Take out the pan from the fridge, release the cake and garnish with the raspberries or strawberries. Slice and serve.

PER SERVING

Cal 985; Fat 62g; Carbs 108g; Protein 9g

Cashew & Cranberry Truffles

Prep time: 5 minutes | Cook time: 15 minutes + chilling time| Serves 4

- 2 cups fresh cranberries
- 2 tbsp pure date syrup
- 1 tsp vanilla extract
- 16 oz coconut cream
- 4 tbsp almond butter
- 3 tbsp cocoa powder
- 2 tbsp pure date sugar

1. Set a silicone egg tray aside. Puree the cranberries, date syrup, and vanilla in a blender until smooth.
2. Add the coconut cream and almond butter to a medium pot over medium heat and simmer the mixture for 2-3 minutes until thoroughly heated, stirring often. Turn the heat off.
3. Mix in the cranberry mixture and divide the mixture into the muffin holes. Refrigerate for 40 minutes or until firm.
4. Remove the tray and pop out the truffles. Nix the cocoa powder and date sugar on a plate. Roll the truffles in the mixture until well dusted and serve.

PER SERVING

Cal 880; Fat 66g; Carbs 64g; Protein 20g

Nutty Date Cake

Prep time: 5 minutes | Cook time:1 hour 30 minutes| Serves 4

- ½ cup cold almond butter, cut into pieces
- 1 egg, beaten
- ½ cup whole-wheat flour
- ¼ cup chopped nuts
- 1 tsp baking powder
- 1 tsp baking soda
- 1 tsp cinnamon powder
- 1 tsp salt
- 1/3 cup dates, chopped
- ½ cup pure date sugar
- 1 tsp vanilla extract
- ¼ cup pure date syrup

1. Preheat your oven to 350°F. In a food processor, add the flour, nuts, baking powder, baking soda, cinnamon powder, and salt. Blend until well combined.
2. Add 1/3 cup of water, almond butter, dates, date sugar, and vanilla. Process until smooth with tiny pieces of dates evident.
3. Pour the batter into a greased baking dish. Bake in the oven for 1 hour and 10 minutes or until a toothpick inserted comes out clean.
4. Remove the dish from the oven, invert the cake onto a serving platter to cool, drizzle with the date syrup, slice, and serve.

PER SERVING

Cal 440; Fat 28g; Carbs 48g; Protein 8g

Mini Chocolate Fudge Squares

Prep time: 5 minutes | Cook time: 20 minutes + chilling time| Serves 6

- 2 cups coconut cream
- 1 tsp vanilla extract
- 3 oz almond butter
- 3 oz dark chocolate

1. Pour coconut cream and vanilla into a saucepan and bring to a boil over medium heat, then simmer until reduced by half, 15 minutes.
2. Stir in almond butter until the batter is smooth. Chop the dark chocolate into bits and stir in the cream until melted.
3. Pour the mixture into a round baking sheet. Chill in the fridge for 3 hours. Serve sliced.

PER SERVING

Cal 445; Fat 44g; Carbs 14g; Protein 4g

Berry Hazelnut Trifle

Prep time: 5 minutes | Cook time: 10 minutes| Serves 4

- 1 ½ ripe avocados
- ¾ cup coconut cream
- ½ lemon, zested and juiced
- 1 tbsp vanilla extract
- 3 oz fresh strawberries
- 2 oz toasted hazelnuts

1. In a bowl, add avocado pulp, coconut cream, lemon zest and juice, and half of the vanilla extract.
2. Mix with an immersion blender. Put the strawberries and remaining vanilla in another bowl and use a fork to mash the fruits.
3. In a tall glass, alternate layering the cream and strawberry mixtures. Drop a few hazelnuts on each and serve.

PER SERVING

Cal 375; Fat 35g; Carbs 14g; Protein 6g

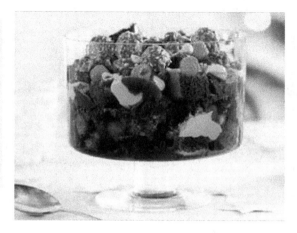

Peanut Chocolate Brownies

Prep time: 5 minutes | Cook time: 40 minutes| Serves 6

- 1 ¾ cups whole-grain flour
- 1 tsp baking powder
- ½ tsp sea salt
- 1 tbsp ground nutmeg
- ½ tsp ground cinnamon
- 3 tbsp cocoa powder
- ½ cup dark chocolate chips
- ½ cup chopped peanuts
- ¼ cup canola oil
- ½ cup dark molasses
- 3 tbsp pure date sugar
- 2 tsp grated fresh ginger

1. Preheat your oven to 360°F. Combine the flour, baking powder, salt, nutmeg, cinnamon, and cocoa in a bowl.
2. Add in chocolate chips and peanuts and stir. Set aside. In another bowl, mix the oil, molasses, ½ cup water, date sugar, and ginger.
3. Pour into the flour mixture and stir to combine. Transfer to a greased baking pan and bake for 30-35 minutes. Let cool before slicing.

PER SERVING

Cal 430; Fat 19g; Carbs 58g; Protein 12g

Chocolate Fudge with Nuts

Prep time: 5 minutes | Cook time: 10 minutes + cooling time| Serves 4

- 3 cups chocolate chips
- ¼ cup thick coconut milk
- 1 ½ tsp vanilla extract
- A pinch of sea salt
- 1 cup chopped mixed nuts

1. Line a square pan with baking paper. Melt the chocolate chips, coconut milk, and vanilla in a medium pot over low heat.
2. Mix in the salt and nuts until well distributed and pour the mixture into the square pan. Refrigerate for at least 2 hours. Cut into squares and serve.

PER SERVING

Cal 905; Fat 32g; Carbs 152g; Protein 8g

Berry Cupcakes with Cashew Cheese Icing

Prep time: 5 minutes | Cook time: 30 minutes + cooling time| Serves 6

- 2 cups whole-wheat flour
- ¼ cup arrowroot
- 2 ½ tsp baking powder
- 1 ½ cups pure date sugar
- ½ tsp salt
- ¾ cup almond butter
- 3 tsp vanilla extract
- 1 cup strawberries, pureed
- 1 cup oat milk
- ¾ cup coconut cream
- 2 tbsp coconut oil, melted
- 3 tbsp pure maple syrup
- 1 tsp vanilla extract
- 1 tsp lemon juice

1. Preheat your oven to 350°F. Line a 12-holed muffin tray with cupcake liners. Set aside. In a bowl, mix flour, arrowroot, baking powder, date sugar, and salt.
2. Whisk in almond butter, vanilla, strawberries, and oat milk until well combined.
3. Divide the mixture into the muffin cups two-thirds way up and bake for 20-25 minutes. Allow cooling while you make the frosting.
4. In a blender, add coconut cream, coconut oil, maple syrup, vanilla, and lemon juice. Process until smooth.
5. Pour the frosting into a medium bowl and chill for 30 minutes. Transfer the mixture into a piping bag and swirl mounds of the frosting onto the cupcakes. Serve.

PER SERVING

Cal 620; Fat 36g; Carbs 72g; Protein 8g

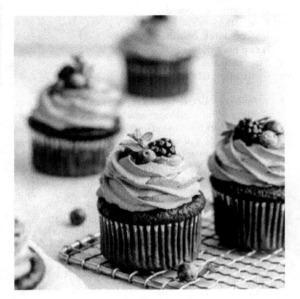

Cinnamon Faux Rice Pudding

Prep time: 5 minutes | Cook time: 25 minutes | Serves 6

- 1 ¼ cups coconut cream
- 1 tsp vanilla extract
- 1 tsp cinnamon powder
- 1 cup mashed tofu
- 2 oz fresh strawberries

1. Pour the coconut cream into a bowl and whisk until a soft peak forms.
2. Mix in the vanilla and cinnamon. Lightly fold in the coconut cream and refrigerate for 10 to 15 minutes to set. Top with the strawberries and serve.

PER SERVING

Cal 215; Fat 19g; Carbs 12g; Protein 4g

Cinnamon Pumpkin Pie

Prep time: 5 minutes | Cook time:70 minutes + cooling time | Serves 4

FOR THE PIECRUST:

- 4 eggs, beaten
- 1/3 cup whole-wheat flour
- ½ tsp salt
- ¼ cup cold almond butter
- 3 tbsp pure malt syrup

FOR THE FILLING:

- ¼ cup pure maple syrup
- ¼ cup pure date sugar
- 1 tsp cinnamon powder
- ½ tsp ginger powder
- 1/8 tsp clove powder
- 1 (15 oz) can pumpkin purée
- 1 cup almond milk

1. Preheat your oven to 350°F. In a bowl, combine flour and salt. Add the almond butter and whisk until crumbly.
2. Pour in crust's eggs, maple syrup, vanilla, and mix until smooth dough forms. Flatten, cover with plastic wrap, and refrigerate for 1 hour.
3. Dust a working surface with flour, remove the dough onto the surface and flatten it into a 1-inch diameter circle. Lay the dough on a greased pie pan and press to fit the shape of the pan.
4. Use a knife to trim the edges of the pan. Lay a parchment paper on the dough, pour on some baking beans and bake for 15-20 minutes. Remove, pour out the baking beans, and allow cooling.
5. In a bowl, whisk the maple syrup, date sugar, cinnamon powder, ginger powder, clove powder, pumpkin puree, and almond milk.
6. Pour the mixture onto the piecrust and bake for 35-40 minutes. Let cool completely. Serve sliced.

PER SERVING

Cal 590; Fat 36g; Carbs 61g; Protein 12g

Mixed Berry Yogurt Ice Pops

Prep time: 5 minutes | Cook time: 5 minutes + chilling time | Serves 6

- 2/3 cup avocado pulp
- 2/3 cup berries
- 1 cup dairy-free yogurt
- ½ cup coconut cream
- 1 tsp vanilla extract

1. Pour the avocado pulp, berries, dairy-free yogurt, coconut cream, and vanilla extract. Process until smooth.
2. Pour into ice pop sleeves and freeze for 8 or more hours. Enjoy the ice pops when ready.

PER SERVING

Cal 145; Fat 12g; Carbs 9g; Protein 3g

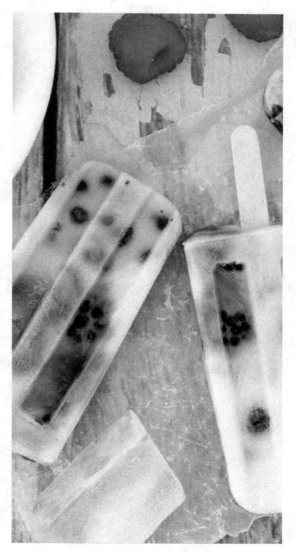

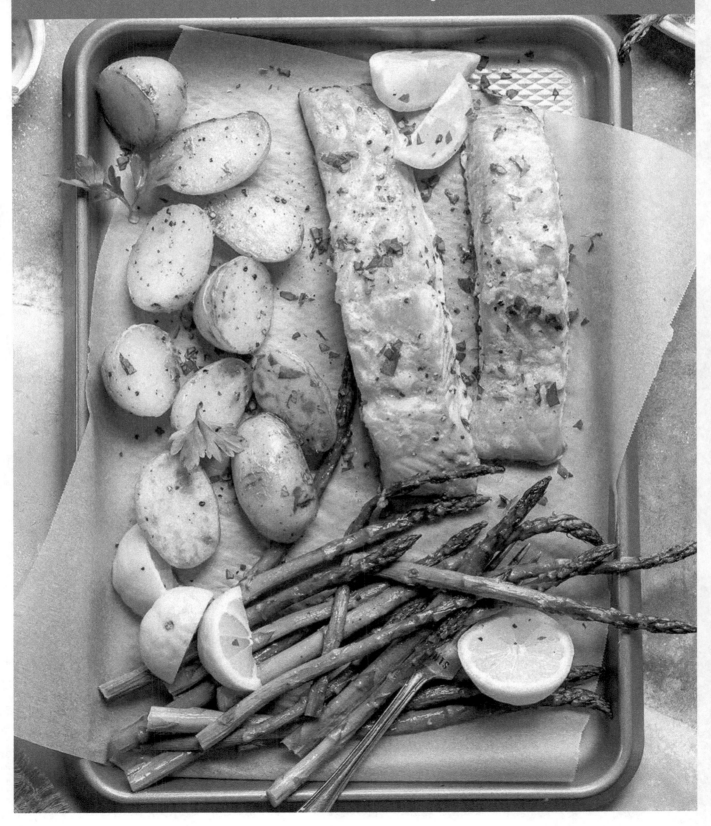

Chapter 16
More Anti-Inflammatory Favorites

Miso Green Cabbage

Prep time: 5 minutes | Cook time: 50 minutes | Serves 4

- 1 lb green cabbage, halved
- 2 tsp olive
- 3 tsp miso paste
- 1 tsp dried oregano
- 1 tbsp balsamic vinegar

1. Preheat your oven to 390°F. Line with parchment paper a baking sheet. Put the green cabbage in a bowl.
2. Coat with olive oil, miso, oregano, rosemary, salt, and pepper. Remove to the baking sheet and bake for 35-40 minutes, shaking every 5 minutes until tender.
3. Remove from the oven to a plate. Drizzle with balsamic vinegar and serve.

PER SERVING

Cal 50; Fat 0.6g; Carbs 10g; Protein 2g

Spicy Steamed Broccoli

Prep time: 5 minutes | Cook time: 15 minutes | Serves 4

- 1 head broccoli, cut into florets
- Sea salt to taste
- 1 tsp red pepper flakes

1. Steam the broccoli florets for 5-7 minutes or until fork-tender.
2. Transfer to a bowl and toss broccoli sprinkle with red pepper flakes and salt. Toss tyo coat. Serve and enjoy!

PER SERVING

Calories: 2; Fat 0g; Carbs: 0.5g; Protein 0.1g

Garlic Roasted Carrots

Prep time: 5 minutes | Cook time: 35 minutes | Serves 4

- 2 lb carrots, cubed
- 2 tsp extra-virgin olive oil
- ½ tsp chili powder
- ½ tsp smoked paprika
- ½ tsp dried oregano
- ½ tsp dried thyme
- ½ tsp garlic powder
- Sea salt to taste

1. Preheat your oven to 400°F. Line with parchment paper a baking sheet. Rinse the carrots and pat dry. Chop into ¾ inch cubes. Place in a bowl and toss with olive oil.
2. In a bowl, mix chili powder, paprika, oregano, thyme, olive oil, salt, and garlic powder. Pour over the carrots and toss to coat.
3. Transfer to a greased baking sheet and bake for 30 minutes, turn once by half. Serve and enjoy!

PER SERVING

Cal 115; Fat 3g; Carbs 22g; Protein 2g

Raisin & Orzo Stuffed Tomatoes

Prep time: 5 minutes | Cook time: 40 minutes | Serves 4

- 2 cups cooked orzo
- Sea salt and pepper to taste
- 3 green onions, minced
- 1/3 cup golden raisins
- 1 tsp orange zest
- 4 large ripe tomatoes
- 1/3 cup toasted pine nuts
- ¼ cup minced fresh parsley
- 2 tsp extra-virgin olive oil

1. Preheat your oven to 380°F. Mix the orzo, green onions, raisins, and orange zest in a bowl. Set aside.
2. Slice the top of the tomato by ½-inch and take out the pulp. Cut the pulp and place it in a bowl. Stir in orzo mixture, pine nuts, parsley, salt, and pepper. Spoon the mixture into the tomatoes and arrange on a greased baking tray.
3. Sprinkle with oil and cover with foil. Bake for 15 minutes. Uncover and bake for another 5 minutes until golden.

PER SERVING

Cal 315; Fat 10g; Carbs 58g; Protein 4g

Eggplant & Hummus Pizza

Prep time: 5 minutes | Cook time: 25 minutes | Serves 2

- ½ eggplant, sliced
- ½ red onion, sliced
- 8 cherry tomatoes, halved
- 3 tbsp chopped black olives
- Sea salt to taste
- Drizzle extra-virgin olive oil
- 2 whole-wheat pizza crusts
- ½ cup hummus
- 2 tbsp oregano

1. Preheat your oven to 390°F. In a bowl, combine the eggplant, onion, tomatoes, olives, and salt. Toss to coat.
2. Sprinkle with some olive oil. Arrange the crusts on a baking sheet and spread the hummus on each pizza. Top with the eggplant mixture. Bake for 20-30 minutes.

PER SERVING

Cal 235; Fat 70g; Carbs 41g; Protein 5g

Steamed Broccoli with Hazelnuts

Prep time: 5 minutes | Cook time: 20 minutes| Serves 4

- ½ cup slivered toasted hazelnuts
- 1 lb broccoli, cut into florets
- 2 tbsp extra-virgin olive oil
- 3 garlic cloves, minced
- 1 cup sliced mushrooms
- ¼ cup dry white wine
- 2 tbsp minced fresh parsley
- Sea salt and pepper to taste

1. Steam the broccoli for 8 minutes or until tender. Remove and set aside. Heat 1 tbsp of oil in a skillet over medium heat.
2. Add garlic and mushrooms and sauté for 5 minutes until tender. Pour in the wine and cook for 1 minute.
3. Stir in broccoli, parsley, salt, and pepper. Cook for 3 minutes until the liquid has reduced.
4. Remove to a bowl and add the remaining oil and hazelnuts; toss to coat. Serve warm.

PER SERVING

Cal 210; Fat 17g; Carbs 12g; Protein 8g

Cilantro Okra

Prep time: 5 minutes | Cook time: 10 minutes| Serves 4

- 2 tbsp extra-virgin olive oil
- 4 cups okra, halved
- Sea salt and pepper to taste
- 3 tbsp chopped cilantro

1. Heat the oil in a skillet over medium heat.
2. Place in the okra, cook for 5 minutes. Turn the heat off and mix in salt, pepper, and cilantro. Serve immediately.

PER SERVING

Cal 95; Fat 7g; Carbs 8g; Protein 2g

Cumin Red & White Cabbage with Apples

Prep time: 5 minutes | Cook time: 30 minutes| Serves 6

- 1 head red cabbage, shredded
- 1 head white cabbage, shredded
- 2 tbsp extra-virgin olive oil
- 1 onion, sliced
- 2 apples, sliced
- 2 tbsp pure date sugar
- ¼ cup cider vinegar
- 1 tsp cumin seeds, crushed
- Sea salt and pepper to taste

1. Heat the oil in a pot over medium heat. Place in onion, shredded cabbages, and apples and sauté for 5 minutes until tender.
2. Stir in date sugar, 1 cup water, vinegar, cumin

seeds, salt, and pepper. Lower the heat and simmer for 20 minutes. Serve right away.

PER SERVING

Cal 145; Fat 5g; Carbs 26g; Protein 4g

Citrus Asparagus

Prep time: 5 minutes | Cook time: 25 minutes| Serves 4

- 1 onion, minced
- 2 tsp lemon zest
- 1/3 cup fresh lemon juice
- 1 tbsp extra-virgin olive oil
- Sea salt and pepper to taste
- 1 lb asparagus, trimmed

1. Combine the onion, lemon zest, lemon juice, and oil in a bowl. Sprinkle with salt and pepper. Let sit for 5-10 minutes.
2. Insert a steamer basket and 1 cup of water in a pot over medium heat.
3. Place the asparagus on the basket and steam for 4-5 minutes until tender but crispy.
4. Leave to cool for 10 minutes, then arrange on a plate. Serve drizzled with the dressing.

PER SERVING

Cal 70; Fat 4g; Carbs 9g; Protein 3g

Japanese-Style Tofu with Haricots Vert

Prep time: 5 minutes | Cook time: 25 minutes| Serves 4

- 5 shiitake mushroom caps, sliced
- 1 cup haricots vert
- 1 tbsp grapeseed oil
- 1 onion, minced
- 1 tsp grated fresh ginger
- 3 green onions, minced
- 8 oz firm tofu, crumbled
- 2 tsp low-sodium soy sauce
- 3 cups hot cooked rice
- 2 tbsp extra-virgin olive oil

1. Place the haricots in boiled salted water and cook for 10 minutes until tender. Drain and set aside. Heat the oil in a skillet over medium heat.
2. Place in onion and cook for 3 minutes until translucent. Add in mushrooms, ginger, green onions, tofu, and soy sauce. Cook for 10 minutes.
3. Share into 4 bowls and top with haricot and tofu mixture. Serve garnished with sesame seeds.

PER SERVING

Cal 495; Fat 34g; Carbs 55g; Protein 22g

Parsley Carrots & Parsnips

Prep time: 5 minutes | Cook time: 25 minutes| Serves 4

- ½ lb carrots, sliced lengthways
- ½ lb parsnips, sliced lengthways
- 2 tbsp extra-virgin olive oil
- Sea salt and pepper to taste
- ½ cup Port wine
- ¼ cup chopped parsley

1. Warm the olive oil in a skillet over medium heat. Place in carrots and parsnips and cook for 5 minutes, stirring occasionally.
2. Sprinkle with salt and pepper. Pour in Port wine and ¼ cup water. Lower the heat and simmer for 15 minutes.
3. Uncover and increase the heat. Cook until a syrupy sauce forms. Serve garnished with parsley.

PER SERVING

Cal 125; Fat 7g; Carbs 15g; Protein 2g

Basil Beet Pasta

Prep time: 5 minutes | Cook time: 20 minutes| Serves 4

- 1 tsp extra-virgin olive oil
- 1 garlic clove, minced
- 4 medium beets, spiralized
- ½ tsp dried basil
- ½ tsp dried oregano
- ½ tsp red pepper flakes

1. Heat the oil in a skillet over medium heat.
2. Place in garlic, beets, basil, oregano, pepper flakes, salt, and pepper. Cook for 15 minutes. Serve and enjoy!

PER SERVING

Cal 50; Fat 1g; Carbs 9g; Protein 5g

Sweet Potatoes with Curry Glaze

Prep time: 5 minutes | Cook time: 20 minutes| Serves 6

- 1 lb sweet potatoes, sliced
- 2 tbsp extra-virgin olive oil
- 2 tbsp curry powder
- 2 tbsp pure date syrup
- Juice of ½ lemon
- Sea salt and pepper to taste

1. Cook the sweet potatoes covered with salted water for 10 minutes. Drain and return them to the pot. Lower the heat.
2. Add oil, curry powder, date syrup, and lemon juice. Cook for 5 minutes. Season with salt and pepper.

PER SERVING

Cal 130; Fat 5g; Carbs 21g; Protein 2g

Date Caramelized Vegetables

Prep time: 5 minutes | Cook time: 30 minutes| Serves 4

- 1 tbsp extra-virgin olive oil
- 2 garlic cloves, minced
- 4 medium shallots, halved
- 3 sweet potatoes, chopped
- 2 large carrots, chopped
- 2 large parsnips, chopped
- 2 small turnips, chopped
- ½ cup pure date sugar
- ¼ cup sherry vinegar
- Sea salt and pepper to taste

1. Heat oil in a skillet over medium heat. Place in garlic and shallots and sauté for 3 minutes. Stir in sweet potatoes, carrots, parsnips, and turnips; cook for 5 minutes until tender.
2. Pour in the sugar, vinegar, and 4 tbsp of water and cook for 5-7 minutes until the sugar dissolves.
3. Season with salt and pepper. Lower the heat and cook for 25 minutes, stirring often.

PER SERVING

Cal 105; Fat 4g; Carbs 28g; Protein 1g

Squash & Zucchini Stir-Fry

Prep time: 5 minutes | Cook time: 20 minutes| Serves 4

- 2 zucchinis, sliced half-moons
- 1 yellow squash, sliced half-moons
- 2 tbsp extra-virgin olive oil
- 1 red onion, sliced
- 3 garlic cloves, sliced
- 1 tsp herbs de Provence

1. Heat oil in a skillet over medium heat. Sauté the onion and garlic for 3 minutes.
2. Mix in zucchini, squash, herbs de Provence, salt, and pepper. Cook for 4-6 minutes, stirring often. Serve and enjoy!

PER SERVING

Cal 70; Fat 7g; Carbs 1g; Protein 0.2g

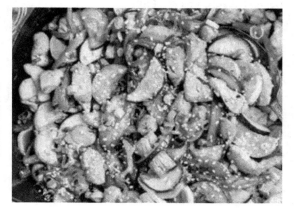

Almond & Chickpea Patties

Prep time: 5 minutes | Cook time: 50 minutes| Serves 6

- 1 roasted red bell pepper, chopped
- 1 (19-oz) can chickpeas
- 1 cup ground almonds
- 2 tsp Dijon mustard
- 2 tsp date syrup
- 1 garlic clove, pressed
- Juice of ½ lemon
- 1 cup kale, chopped
- 1½ cups rolled oats

1. Preheat your oven to 360°F. In a blender, place the chickpeas, almonds, bell pepper, mustard, date syrup, garlic, lemon juice, and kale. Pulse until ingredients are finely chopped but not over blended.
2. Add in the oats. Pulse until everything is well combined. Shape the mixture into 12 patties and arrange on a greased baking sheet.
3. Bake for 30 minutes until light brown. Serve.

PER SERVING

Cal 225; Fat 11g; Carbs 32g; Protein 8g

Spaghetti Squash in Tahini Sauce

Prep time: 5 minutes | Cook time: 50 minutes| Serves 4

- 1 (3-pound) spaghetti squash, halved lengthwise
- 1 tbsp rice vinegar
- 1 tbsp tahini
- Sea salt and pepper to taste

1. Preheat your oven to 390°F. Line with wax paper a baking sheet. Slice the squash half lengthwise and arrange on the baking sheet skin-side up.
2. Bake for 35-40 minutes. Let cool before scraping the flesh to make "noodles."
3. Place the spaghetti in a bowl. In another bowl, whisk 1 tbsp hot water, vinegar, tahini, salt, and pepper.
4. Add into the spaghetti bowl and toss to coat. Serve and enjoy!

PER SERVING

Cal 70; Fat 2g; Carbs 12g; Protein 2g

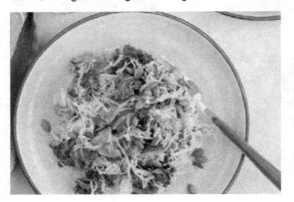

Sherry Eggplants with Cherry Tomatoes

Prep time: 5 minutes | Cook time: 20 minutes| Serves 4

- 1 garlic cloves, minced
- 2 tbsp tamari sauce
- 1 tbsp dry sherry
- 1 tsp extra-virgin olive oil
- ½ tsp pure date sugar
- 1 tbsp canola oil
- 2 unpeeled eggplants, sliced
- 2 green onions, minced
- 10 black olives, chopped

1. Combine the garlic, tamari, sherry, olive oil, and sugar in a bowl. Set aside. Heat the oil in a skillet over medium heat.
2. Place in the eggplant slices, fry for 4 minutes per side. Spread the tamari sauce on the eggplants.
3. Pour in ¼ cup water and cook for 15 minutes. Remove to a plate and sprinkle with green onions and black olives. Serve.

PER SERVING

Cal 130; Fat 6g; Carbs 19g; Protein 3g

Maple Green Cabbage Hash

Prep time: 5 minutes | Cook time: 25 minutes| Serves 4

- 3 tbsp extra-virgin olive oil
- 2 shallots, thinly sliced
- 1 lb green cabbage, grated
- 3 tbsp apple cider vinegar
- 1 tbsp pure maple syrup
- ½ tsp sriracha sauce

1. Heat the oil in a skillet over medium heat. Place in shallots and cabbage and cook for 10 minutes until tender.
2. Pour in vinegar and scrape any bits from the bottom.
3. Mix in maple syrup and sriracha sauce. Cook for 3-5 minutes until the liquid absorbs. Sprinkle with salt and pepper.

PER SERVING

Cal 175; Fat 13g; Carbs 13g; Protein 2g

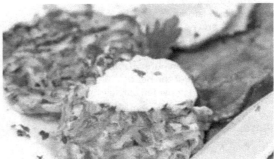

Peanut Quinoa & Chickpea Pilaf

Prep time: 5 minutes | Cook time: 30 minutes| Serves 4

- 1 tbsp extra-virgin olive oil
- 1 red onion, minced
- 1 ½ cups quinoa, rinsed
- 3 cups vegetable broth
- 2 (15.5-oz) cans chickpeas
- ¼ tsp ground cayenne
- 1 tbsp minced fresh chives
- 1 tangerine, chopped
- ½ cup peanuts

1. Heat the oil in a pot over medium heat. Place the onion and cook for 3 minutes until softened.
2. Add in quinoa and broth. Bring to a boil, then lower the heat and sprinkle with salt.
3. Simmer for 20 minutes. Stir in chickpeas, cayenne pepper, chives, tangerine, and peanuts. Serve.

PER SERVING

Cal 580; Fat 20g; Carbs 80g; Protein 28g

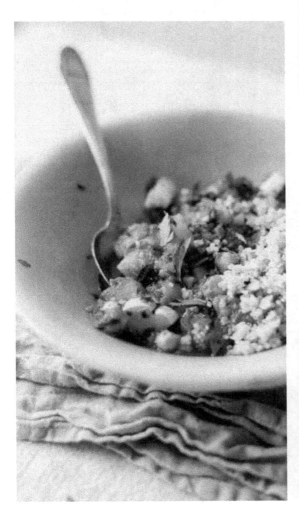

Korean-Style Buckwheat

Prep time: 5 minutes | Cook time: 25 minutes| Serves 4

- 1 cup buckwheat groats
- ¼ cup rice vinegar
- ¼ cup Mirin wine

1. Boil 2 cups of water in a pot. Put in the buckwheat groats, lower the heat, and simmer covered for 15-20 minutes until the liquid absorbs.
2. Let cool for a few minutes. Fluff the groats and stir in vinegar and Mirin wine. Serve.

PER SERVING

Cal 45; Fat 0.5g; Carbs 9g; Protein 2g

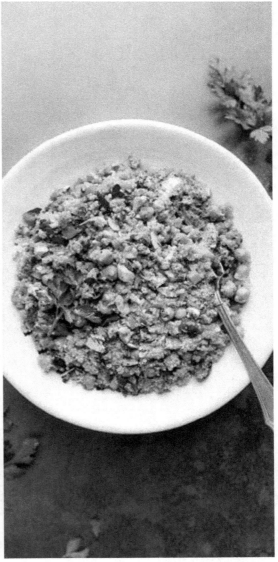

Appendix 1 Measurement Conversion Chart

Volume Equivalents (Dry)

US STANDARD	METRIC (APPROXIMATE)
1/8 teaspoon	0.5 mL
1/4 teaspoon	1 mL
1/2 teaspoon	2 mL
3/4 teaspoon	4 mL
1 teaspoon	5 mL
1 tablespoon	15 mL
1/4 cup	59 mL
1/2 cup	118 mL
3/4 cup	177 mL
1 cup	235 mL
2 cups	475 mL
3 cups	700 mL
4 cups	1 L

Volume Equivalents (Liquid)

US STANDARD	US STANDARD (OUNCES)	METRIC (APPROXIMATE)
2 tablespoons	1 fl.oz.	30 mL
1/4 cup	2 fl.oz.	60 mL
1/2 cup	4 fl.oz.	120 mL
1 cup	8 fl.oz.	240 mL
1 1/2 cup	12 fl.oz.	355 mL
2 cups or 1 pint	16 fl.oz.	475 mL
4 cups or 1 quart	32 fl.oz.	1 L
1 gallon	128 fl.oz.	4 L

Temperatures Equivalents

FAHRENHEIT(F)	CELSIUS(C) APPROXIMATE
225 °F	107 °C
250 °F	120 ° °C
275 °F	135 °C
300 °F	150 °C
325 °F	160 °C
350 °F	180 °C
375 °F	190 °C
400 °F	205 °C
425 °F	220 °C
450 °F	235 °C
475 °F	245 °C
500 °F	260 °C

Weight Equivalents

US STANDARD	METRIC (APPROXIMATE)
1 ounce	28 g
2 ounces	57 g
5 ounces	142 g
10 ounces	284 g
15 ounces	425 g
16 ounces (1 pound)	455 g
1.5 pounds	680 g
2 pounds	907 g

Appendix 2 The Dirty Dozen and Clean Fifteen

The Environmental Working Group (EWG) is a nonprofit, nonpartisan organization dedicated to protecting human health and the environment Its mission is to empower people to live healthier lives in a healthier environment. This organization publishes an annual list of the twelve kinds of produce, in sequence, that have the highest amount of pesticide residue-the Dirty Dozen-as well as a list of the fifteen kinds ofproduce that have the least amount of pesticide residue-the Clean Fifteen.

THE DIRTY DOZEN	
The 2016 Dirty Dozen includes the following produce. These are considered among the year's most important produce to buy organic:	
Strawberries	Spinach
Apples	Tomatoes
Nectarines	Bell peppers
Peaches	Cherry tomatoes
Celery	Cucumbers
Grapes	Kale/collard greens
Cherries	Hot peppers

The Dirty Dozen list contains two additional itemskale/ collard greens and hot peppers-because they tend to contain trace levels of highly hazardous pesticides.

THE CLEAN FIFTEEN	
The least critical to buy organically are the Clean Fifteen list. The following are on the 2016 list:	
Avocados	Papayas
Corn	Kiw
Pineapples	Eggplant
Cabbage	Honeydew
Sweet peas	Grapefruit
Onions	Cantaloupe
Asparagus	Cauliflower
Mangos	

Some of the sweet corn sold in the United States are made from genetically engineered (GE) seedstock. Buy organic varieties of these crops to avoid GE produce.

Appendix 3 Index

GRACE K. LAWS

CPSIA information can be obtained
at www.ICGtesting.com
Printed in the USA
LVHW060836201122
733283LV00012B/383

9 781739 180577